The European Union and Health Policy

Ed Randall
Lecturer in Social Policy and Politics
Goldsmiths College
University of London

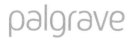

© Ed Randall 2001

First published 2001 by
PALGRAVE
Houndmills, Basingstoke, Hampshire RG21 6XS and
175 Fifth Avenue, New York, N. Y. 10010
Companies and representatives throughout the world

PALGRAVE is the new global academic imprint of
St. Martin's Press LLC Scholarly and Reference Division and
Palgrave Publishers Ltd (formerly Macmillan Press Ltd).

ISBN 0–333–75426–3

This book is printed on paper suitable for recycling and
made from fully managed and sustained forest sources.

A catalogue record for this book is available
from the British Library.

Library of Congress Cataloging-in-Publication Data
Randall, Ed, 1951–
    The European union and health policy / Ed Randall.
        p. cm.
    Includes bibliographical references and index.
    ISBN 0–333–75426–3
    1. Public health—European Union countries. 2. Medical policy–
    –European Union countries. 3. Health planning—European Union
    countries. I. Title.

RA483 .R36 2000
362.1'094—dc21
                                                        00–034490

10   9   8   7   6   5   4   3   2   1
10   09 08 07 06 05 04 03 02 01

Printed and bound in Great Britain by
Antony Rowe Ltd, Chippenham, Wiltshire

For Jane and Ted, Elizabeth and Rachel and Nancy

Contents

List of Tables, Figures and Boxes

Tables

Figures

Boxes

Preface

This book is about the developing and growing involvement of the European Union (EU) in health policy. The Treaties of Maastricht and Amsterdam require the EU to take the health of European citizens very seriously and to consider health in all that the EU does. Although the EU has no direct involvement in the delivery of health services in member states its range of responsibilities, including the ramifications, for health, of the Single European Market (SEM) and its specific competence in the field of public health, make it a major player in European health policy. The lack of a direct responsibility for the management of health-care systems may explain why the academic literature on European health policy appears so thin, when compared with what has been written about other areas of EU responsibility and activity. Given the importance of, and interest in, health issues in the EU and the EU's role in tackling threats to health, I am nevertheless a little shocked to have to report that this is the first major political study solely devoted to the subject.

The European Commission's response to BSE demonstrated both Commission powers and weaknesses. The Commission and the Union were greatly affected by the Bovine Spongiform Encephalopathy (BSE) crisis. Work on health in the Commission has been reorganised and is now managed by the newly created Commission Directorate of Health and Consumer Protection, a development that undoubtedly reflects the political sensitivity and political prominence gained by health issues in the 1990s. Change, in a Union where the lives of citizens are becoming ever more closely linked together, economically and politically, can be rapid and sometimes, as with BSE, unexpected – even though the instruments of European policy-making seem ill-equipped to make anything happen quickly. In the course of writing this book I have been made aware of just how quickly the political and policy landscape can change in Europe. The mass resignation of the Commission in March 1999 was an event that few commentators predicted and the Prodi Commission has recently promised a pace of change and reform in the Commission that has also taken many observers by surprise. Readers of this book, which is designed to provide the most complete and up-to-date account of the EU role in health and health-related policy – for the start of the new millennium – will be aware that the book's subject does not stand still. Fortunately the account of EU health and health related policy provided here can easily be supplemented by making use of the rapidly expanding internet resources being developed by the European Commission and the European Agencies, which feature extensively in this book.

Good health is fundamental to the quality of all our lives – a fact that is reflected in the value most of us place on our own and other people's health. This high valuation is mirrored in the considerable resources we are prepared to put into health services, as taxpayers and as private consumers. But health services are generally called upon when health is failing or compromised in some fashion – when improving or protecting health is most difficult. One of the key messages from the Union's health-policy-makers and from health-policy specialists, located in member states and international organisations, is that health policy needs to be fully integrated into both economic and social policy to ensure that health can be more efficiently and effectively promoted and protected. A vital ingredient for such integration is international co-operation. This book is, above all else, an account of European collaboration in the field of health and an exploration of the case for strengthening existing collaborations so that health issues can be better integrated into all that the EU does.

ED RANDALL

Acknowledgements

I would like to thank all the people who helped me and may have wondered if this book would ever be completed. Many people who have helped me and worked with me over the years may not know that they have made a contribution to this book but they have; it would simply be impractical to list them all. Tony Butcher and Tim Newburn read through drafts of each chapter and their friendly reception of each chapter provided me with the encouragement to keep going. Shirley Angel and Barbara Boon understood when I was unable to be the kind of colleague that they deserve. The Library of the King's Fund was an invaluable resource and I am grateful to the staff there: they are always helpful and welcoming. I have also made extensive use of material that is only available on the world wide web. My admiration and appreciation for the skills of web designers, most especially those who work on the web pages of the European Commission, continues to grow.

My greatest thanks must go to my wife and my daughter who have had a lot to put up with while I have been working on *The European Union and Health Policy*. I owe a particular debt to my father and I am very grateful for his support and encouragement and for my mother-in-law's help; they have both been more helpful in this enterprise than they can know.

List of Abbreviations

ACSHH	Advisory Committee for Safety, Hygiene and Health Protection at Work
AIDS	Acquired Immune Deficiency Syndrome
AIM	Advanced Informatics in Medicine
ASPHER	Association of Schools of Public Health in the European Region
BIOMED	Biomedical and Health Research Programme of the EU
BMJ	*British Medical Journal*
BSE	Bovine Spongiform Encephalopathy
CAP	Common Agricultural Policy
CEEC	Central and Eastern European Countries
CELAD	The European Committee to Combat Drugs
CEN	Comité Européen de Normalisation
CEPHCP	(European Parliament's) Committee for Environment, Public Health and Consumer Protection
CJD/vCJD/nvCJD	Creutzfeldt Jacob Disease/variant/new variant
COREPER	Committee of Permanent Representatives
DG III	Commission Directorate responsible for Industrial Affairs
DG V	Directorate General Five (Employment and Social Affairs)
DG XXIV	Consumer Protection Directorate of the European Commission
EAEC	European Atomic Energy Community (see Euratom)
EASHW	European Agency for Safety and Health at Work
EC	European Community
ECHR	European Convention on Human Rights
ECJ	European Court of Justice
ECSC	European Coal and Steel Community
Ecu	European Currency Unit
EEA	European Economic Area
EEC	European Economic Community(ies)
EFILWC	European Foundation for the Improvement of Living and Working Conditions
EHLASS	European Home and Leisure Accidents Surveillance System Programme

EIB	European Investment Bank
EIU	Economist Intelligent Unit
EMCDDA	European Monitoring Centre for Drugs and Drug Addiction
EMDIS	European Marrow Donor Information System
EMEA	European Agency for the Evaluation of Medicinal Products
EMU	European Monetary Union
EP	European Parliament
EPHA	European Public Health Alliance
ERDF	European Regional Development Fund
ESAW	European Statistics on Accidents at Work
ESC	Economic and Social Committee
ESF	European Social Fund
ETHOS	European Telematics Horizontal Observatory Service
EU	European Union
Euratom	European Atomic Energy Community (see EAEC)
Euro	Common European currency
EURES	European Employment Services
EUROSTAT	Statistical Office of the European Communities
EWON	European Network on Work Organisation
FP5	Fifth Framework Programme for research
GDP	Gross Domestic Product
GNP	Gross National Product
HDSE	Human Dignity and Social Exclusion project
HFA	Health For All (World Health Organisation)
HIEMS	Health Indicators Exchange and Monitoring System
HIV	Human Immunodeficiency Virus
HSSCD	Health Surveillance System for Communicable Diseases
ICH	International Conference on Harmonisation
ICT	Information and Communications Technology(ies)
IDA	Interchange of Data between Administrations
IGC	Intergovernmental Conference
ISPO	Information Society Project Office
ISTAHC	International Society of Technology Assessment in Health Care
MAFF	The Ministry of Agriculture Food and Fisheries
MHR	Medical and Health Research Programme
MINE	Medicines Information Network for Europe
MRAs	Mutual Recognition Agreements

OECD	Organisation for Economic Co-operation and Development
OELs	Occupational Exposure Limits
OHE	Office of Health Economics
OJ	*Official Journal of the European Communities*
OSH	Occupational Safety and Health
QMV	Qualified Majority Voting
R&D	Research and Development
R&TD	Research and Technological Development
REITOX	The European Information Network on Drugs and Drug Addiction
SBO	Specified Bovine Offal
SCADPLUS	EU's web-based guide to its policies
SCOEL	Scientific Committee on Occupational Exposure Limits
SEA	Single European Act
SEAC	Spongiform Encepalopathy Advisory Committee
SEG	Scientific Expert Group
SEM	Single European Market
SLIC	Senior Labour Inspectors' Committee
SLIM	Simpler Legislation for the Internal Market
SMEs	Small and Medium-Sized Enterprises
TEU	Treaty on EU
TSEs	Transmissable Spongiform Encephalopathies
WHO	World Health Organisation

PART I

The European Communities' Developing Role in Health

1
Introduction: the EC/EU and Health Policy

Political projects, ambitions and opportunities

Few could have envisaged the way in which the creation of the European Coal and Steel Community (ECSC) in 1951, by the Treaty of Paris, would lead on to five decades of European institution building and European policy-making. Those adults who, now aged over 60, dreamt in 1950 of a Europe in which warring nation states counted for much less and the common interests of ordinary Europeans counted for a great deal more, may be disappointed with the state of the EU at the end of the 20th century. But they might – nevertheless – feel some satisfaction at what European co-operation has achieved and permit themselves some optimism about where it is leading. It is a long way from constructing an organisation designed to build and sustain economic integration – in coal and steel production – to a pan-European political framework and institutional apparatus which, among many many other things, seeks to make and influence health policy for almost all of Western Europe's democracies.

Michael Maclay writes of one of the two men responsible for the establishment of the ECSC, Jean Monnet, that he was: '. . . a man who understood varieties of nations and nationhood . . . [whose] . . . experience pointed him to the belief that nations would do their people most proud when they found ways of pooling their strengths' (1998: 13). Monnet not only believed that the whole could be stronger than the sum of its parts – but he also believed passionately that realising the potential of the whole depended upon taking small but effective steps, which had clear practical value and obvious rewards, for as many of the collaborators as possible. For Monnet and Schumann the establishment of the ECSC was 'a limited but decisive point' and for Monnet, in particular, it was pregnant with possibilities for healing and uniting Europe. Schumann

3

said of Europe: '. . . [it] will not be built at a stroke, nor constructed in accordance with some overall plan: it will be built upon concrete achievements which first create a *de facto* solidarity' (Bainbridge with Teasdale 1995: 401). He was expressing a belief in the efficacy of modest actions enabling nations and citizens to learn more about each other and to discover what they can achieve together. The account of the EU and health policy offered in this book is consistent with the view that modest achievements often lead on to greater things.

While an appreciation of the potential and relevance that political and social ideals have is vitally important, in making sense of European institutions and policies, an appreciation of the practical and institutional details of European policy-making is also necessary. It calls for an understanding of the extent to which successful institution building and policy formulation depends on the ingenuity, resourcefulness and determination of individual human beings, often public servants – both elected and unelected. Monnet was, like another great social and political architect mentioned below, William Beveridge, a British civil servant for a time. Later, as head of the French *Commisariat du Plan*, he found a politician, Robert Schuman, with whom he was able to collaborate closely. Such collaborations are often of great importance in policy-making and institution-building, but they are also often poorly reported (for an exception see Maclay, 1998: 30).

The complex structure of the EU and its institutions means – as this book seeks to show – that the quality of relationships between public servants can be even more critical at European level than it is at national level, in transforming policy proposals and ideas into practical schemes of action (Ross, 1995: 26–39; El-Agraa, 1998: 36). Monnet's belief in and enthusiasm for practical steps contrasts with the idealism of the Italian federalist leader, another architect of modern Europe, Altiero Spinelli (1907–86), whose European aspirations were reflected in plans and proposals to create a popular constituent assembly in which representatives from across Europe could formulate a European constitution and form a European polity (Pinder, 1998: 5). Monnet's success in laying institutional foundations was a necessary – if not sufficient – condition for the elected European Parliament, which Spinelli joined in 1979, following the first Europe-wide election for the Parliament. Finding and then building on things that could be agreed between nation states, rather than challenging nation states directly was an essential part of Monnet's approach to European integration.

Monnet's approach not only contrasts with that of Spinelli but it can also be contrasted with the British approach to planning and founding its welfare state. William Beveridge offered the British people a blueprint for social advance and a modern caring state – a state that could provide for its citizens from cradle to grave. Beveridge's grand plans and his presentation of them, which closely linked economic and social policy, have arguably acted as a powerful constraint on re-formulating and reinvigorating the social purposes which Beveridge saw himself – along with many others – as serving (Glennerster, 1995: 1–42). Monnet's aspirational – yet practical and circumspect – approach to the formulation of social and economic institutions, has arguably stood the test of time rather better than the detailed, but ultimately less ambitious, approach to planning for the future adopted in Britain during and immediately after the Second World War.

The great ambition, which underpinned Monnet and Schumann's proposal for the ECSC, cannot be in doubt. It was recognised by political leaders of their day. Although the European Economic Community (EEC), which was built upon the success of the ECSC, has often been presented in Britain as little more than a free trade zone astute political leaders understood that it and the ECSC before it were much more than that. The need for political and social co-operation – as well as economic integration – was part of the *raison d'être* of those, including Monnet and Schumann, who argued that the Schuman Declaration of 9 May 1950 represented 'concrete steps... to the preservation of peace' (Schuman Declaration, 1950). When he resigned as President of the High Authority, the forerunner to the present day European Commission, Monnet established an Action Committee for a United States of Europe which worked steadfastly to extend and promote his European project (Bainbridge, with Teasdale 1995: 335; Ross, 1995: 246: Pinder, 1998: 143–145). The title of the organisation left little doubt about the kind of European integration that Monnet sought.

While they may not have had a detailed route map, Schuman and Monnet did have politically intoxicating ideas about what European collaboration could and should lead on to. A leading British politician, Harold Macmillan, who recognised and had some qualified sympathy with their vision, commenting on the Schuman Plan, observed that: 'To the great majority of Europeans, by far the most significant aspect of M. Schuman's initiative is the political. It is not, in its essentials, a purely economic or industrial conception; it is a grand design for a new Europe; it is not just a piece of convenient machinery; it is a revolutionary, almost mystical conception' (Bainbridge with Teasdale, 1995: 401). In similar vein Konrad Adenaur told the Bundestag in 1952 that the political import of the ECSC was '. . . infinitely larger than its economic purpose. . . . For the first time in history, countries want to renounce part of their sovereignty, voluntarily and without compulsion, in order to transfer it to a supranational structure' (Bainbridge with Teasdale, 1995: 159).

Judged against such dramatic and rhetorical language the political achievements of European political institutions may appear somewhat underwhelming. Monnet was attracted by a vision of European political institutions that was capable of improving the lives of Europeans, irrespective of their national identity, in the most practical ways possible. He wanted those institutions to be built co-operatively by Germany and France – and as many other European nations as could be involved. Britain's unwillingness to become involved was a particular disappointment. British politicians rejected, for many years, what they feared was an integrationist brew, fermented by Monnet and others, to extinguish British identity and independence. Many British political leaders still suspect a deep plot to deprive the British of their historical uniqueness and independence.

British political leaders specifically rejected the ECSC and later on the EEC (as well as the European Atomic Energy Community (EAEC or EURATOM)). For many years the states which formed the EEC and EAEC themselves seemed satisfied to focus on the economic benefits and aims of the treaties they had signed. Despite that – and it is a core argument of this book – a process of social and political begetting had been started which has demonstrably done more than maintain the peace between member states and contribute to their economic success in the latter half of the 20th century.

Among the capabilities which European institutions have acquired is a capability to shape and formulate policies that affect the health of the people of Europe. The idea that significant contributions to health can come from policy measures which do not bear directly on the delivery of health services has been a vital ingredient in this. It helps to explain the willingness of European political leaders and policy-makers to support a role for the EU in health and health-related policy-making (Belcher, 1997a: 1–3). It is possible, however, that a powerful genie has been released that will not be returned to its bottle.

Spill over

Wise and Gibb (1993) in their *Single Market to Social Europe – the European Community in the 1990s*, make much of the idea of 'spill over'. In doing so they refer to a theory which 'has permeated much of the academic literature on the process of European unity' (33). In essence their approach relies on the idea that even limited economic, social or political co-operation and integration can build-up pressures to co-operate and integrate across an increasing number of related policy areas. Given the extent of economic co-operation envisaged in the Treaties of Paris and of Rome spill over implies that the removal or absence of controls on economic exchange between nation states fosters calls for policies which help to manage the unwanted side-effects of economic competition and free capital movements. Observers of the EEC – and now the EU – have pointed to the existence of regional policies and structural funds as evidence of spill over effects from trade liberalisation and of a willingness to recognise and respond to them collectively. The spill over approach implies that a political corollary of increasing economic competition is a willingness to address and resolve questions of unfairness; even if protestations of unfairness are made without evidence of obvious damage or of unwanted side-effects. A sense of injustice can be a strong motivating factor on its own. In contemporary language spill over can be politically significant whenever and wherever there is an acceptance of the need to create or maintain 'a level playing field'.

If a commitment to open economic competition amongst nations is based on a set of agreed rules and on common understandings, then a willingness to resolve disputes and support agreed arrangements for resolving disputes is vital. It becomes a fundamental requirement for continued co-operation between partners. It seems reasonable to assume that people who share many of the same ideas about democratic institutions and economic competition and jurisprudence can, with a little goodwill – and in the absence of fundamental differences in their interests, develop effective ways of dealing with spill over issues and effects. Wise and Gibb take the view that 'practical people, concerned with the changing political shape of Europe', have always subscribed to the tenets of spill over and include – 'most notably . . . Jean Monnet and Robert Schuman' (1993: 34).

In his memoirs Jean Monnet made clear his view that developing interrelationships between nation states would ultimately and necessarily lead to stronger supranational institutions:

> the Community we have created is not an end in itself. . . . It is a process of change . . . our nations today must learn to live together under common rules and institutions freely arrived at. The sovereign nations of the past can no longer solve the problems of the present: they cannot ensure their own progress or control their own future.
>
> (Fontaine, 1994: 6)

A broader vision and the public health

The authors and advocates of *the new public health* and others who organise to protect the environment and talk of the need to think globally and act locally appear to share Jean Monnet's views about the importance of reforming political institutions and looking beyond the nation state (MacDonald, 1998: 24–25, 28–30). Spill over and the impotence of nation states, in the face of health scourges, environmental pollution and economic and social change, provide much of the background to the discussion of European health and health-related policy in this book. The new public health is based on a view of public health activism that sees little distinction between health policy and public policy as a whole.

The new public health has been described as, 'at its core a moral enterprise, in that it involves prescriptions about how we should live our lives individually and collectively' (Petersen, 1996: xii). It is an approach to health which, much like Monnet's plans for Europe (Fontaine, 1994, 12), rests on a great optimism about professionalism, disinterested science and 'rational administrative solutions to problems' (Petersen, 1996: xii). In its *Alma Ata Declaration,* made in 1987, the World Health Organisation (WHO) asserted that 'the attainment of the highest possible level of health is a most important world-wide social goal whose realization requires the action of many other social and economic sectors in addition to the health sector' (WHO, 1978: Para 1). The WHO has since been responsible for a series of ringing declarations about the relationship between environment and health and the importance, for health, of achieving social justice. The declarations and statements include the: the *Ottawa Charter* (1986), The European Charter on Environment and Health (1989), The Milan Declaration on Healthy Cities (1990), Helsinki Declaration on Action for the Environment and Health in Europe (1994a), The Copenhagen Declaration (1994b), The Ljubljana Charter on Reforming Health Care (1996) and The Athens Declaration for Healthy Cities (1998a). The essential message remains the same: 'Key principles for health [are] equity . . . sustainability . . . intersectoral collaboration [and] . . . solidarity' (WHO, 1998a: Paras 1–4).

The passion and zeal of those who subscribe most strongly to the new public health can be a little frightening. Petersen and Lupton make much of the ways in which the new public health provides a social and political space in which the contemporary state can claim authority over individuals and communities (1996: 174–81). Few if any aspects of our human existence are off limits and few, if any, areas of public policy are – from the perspective of the new public health – unrelated to health concerns. As Petersen and Lupton put it: . . . 'there is a new consciousness of risks that are believed to lie beyond the individual's control but which are viewed as, ultimately, a result of human activity' (1996: 1). They go on to list, as examples of the multitude of environmental factors which arouse the anxieties of citizens of the world's most developed states, hazardous chemicals, global warming and the loss of biodiversity. And they note, as they do so, that the greatest anxieties about environmental and other modern risks are linked to concerns about human health. Indeed the fecund, in a political sense, territory with which the proponents of the new public health wish to deal raises numerous questions about individuals and individual responsibilities for health. The expertise and skills of health policy-makers can be directed not only at influencing the actions of governments – they can also be (and frequently are) directed at the ways in which individuals live their lives and care for themselves and their immediate environment. In striking language Petersen and Lupton characterise concern with the 'healthy body', promoted by the new public health, as a modern fashion on which image entrepreneurs of all kinds (and that includes health policy-makers) can play and contrast it with the *old* public health. Petersen and Lupton write that: 'While the "old" public health strategies focused almost entirely on issues of public hygiene – the cleanliness of the streets, sanitation and water supply – the new public health has directed its attention towards the conduct and appearance of the individual body' (1996: 23). There is, as they point out, a certain open-endedness about health promotion, health education and health improvement pro-grammes and – for that reason – a legitimate concern about the role of the experts and insiders who drive and shape public policies intended to improve and protect the health of the public. Concern which they suggest should be heightened by the new public health strategist's determination to enlist the whole of the population in a great variety of health projects covering virtually every aspect of daily living.

The tone and language employed by Petersen and Lupton suggests the possibility of sinister goings on. Is it possible that public health concerns may act as a cover for unhealthy (at least in a political sense) developments in the relationship between the modern state and its citizens? It is a possibility that should not be overlooked or ignored; but it is a possibility that needs to be considered in a balanced way. The influence sought by the EU Commission, through its health projects and policies, and its scope for action may appear substantial – if poorly funded. But there are also very substantial impediments to the forward march of the new public health, apart from limited funding.

John Ashton and Howard Seymour identify some of the many factors that impede and qualify the onward march of professionals and experts concerned with the public health (1988: 84–85). Those factors have been the everyday concerns of health-policy makers working for the European Commission's Directorate General Five (DGV). It has, until very recently, had the major responsibility for managing the work associated with the EU's public health competence.

Ashton and Seymour describe the 'dilemmas' which face practitioners of health promotion. In doing so they are also describing the very real limitations and constraints which affect almost all public health programmes and projects, especially those which lack clear public support. Health promoters, however enthusiastic, quickly find out that health is rarely under their direct influence. As Ashton and Seymour put it: 'Health is gained, lost and maintained in the real world of work, home, leisure and daily life'. Unless the concerns of health promoters coincide with those of the individuals – with whose health they are concerned – health promoters face an uphill battle in the 'real world . . . of daily life'. The professionals and experts who wish to act as guides and educators to others live in an age when respect for them and what they have to say is qualified – not least because experts are in direct competition with many other would be persuaders. 'Traditional health educators', in Ashton's and Seymour's words, 'can have a relatively small impact on people during most of their lives' (1998: 84). The lengthy and far from successful battle that health promoters, educators and policy-makers have waged against tobacco products is clear and persuasive testimony, if any were needed, that being knowledgeable and well-intentioned is not enough. The experts have generally failed to capture the attention of the young or to exert a lasting influence over the behaviour of millions of smokers.

The difficulties encountered by would be health promoters and health educators do not end with the problems they meet in getting the public's attention or in gaining access to other people's lives. In practice the proponents of the new public health have had modest success in challenging the priorities and shifting the attention of elected policy-makers and political leaders from expensive institutional health services. Despite several decades of eloquent and highly respectable scientific argument from epidemiologists it remains the case that public resources for health care are concentrated on sickness services and that there has been little shift in public expenditure towards health promotion and illness prevention work. Inpatient services consume most health service resources; between 45 per cent and 75 per cent of health care resources (McKeown, 1976; Saltman and Figueras, 1997: 217).

The modest impact of the new public health on public policy reflects another fact of contemporary political life – the intensity of competition for tax revenues and public resources. Indeed the productivity of the new public health, in terms of politically controversial and difficult proposals – and the vastness of the policy agendas it promotes, make it deeply unattractive to many elected representatives. Political leaders, who have to balance general health and environmental concerns against the exigencies of managing limited budgets, are understandably wary about public health issues and concerns.

Assailed by rising expectations for health services of all kinds it is easy to understand why those who seek election, and have a realistic prospect of winning office, approach grand proposals for designing a healthier society very cautiously. Welcoming 'good ideas' while promoting the greatest possible economy in the use of public revenues is surely the most sensible stratagem, for those who wish to be elected and re-elected. Public health zealots can – with some justification – be told 'you don't have to stand for election'. One of the great contemporary political conundrums is how to communicate enthusiasm for the kinds of health targets promoted by bodies such as the WHO and – at the same time – keep demands for additional resources and powers in check. It is a conundrum to which there is unlikely to be a truly satisfactory political solution.

The *Health For All* (HFA) strategy of the WHO, set out in WHO's *Global Strategy for Health for All by the Year 2000* (WHO, 1981), was an inspiring – Monnet like – statement of common purpose in the field of health. Its grand ambitions were a product of the intellectual and political excitement kindled by a broader vision of the public health. HFA called on governments around the world to make their main social target the 'attainment by all citizens of the world by the year 2000 a level of health that will permit them to lead socially and economically productive [lives]'. The statement was widely adopted and supported; in the UK, for example, *Health of the Nation* policies and publications were promoted strongly by both Conservative and Labour administrations. The European Regional Committee of WHO developed a strategy for Europe, with a large number of specific health targets, which was adopted by member states in 1985; the very same states that make up the membership of the EU.

The themes embodied in HFA reflect one of the most remarkable – and some would say unrealistic – definitions of health ever propounded. A definition of health that can serve as a back-cloth to health and health-related policy-making in the EU. The WHO defined health, in 1948, as 'a state of complete physical, social and mental well-being and not merely the absence of disease or infirmity'.

In its *Health in Europe – 1997 Report on the Third Evaluation of Progress Towards Health for All in the European Region of WHO*, WHO assesses progress in achieving health outcomes and specific health targets. It does so in terms of what it describes as 'the four cornerstones of the HFA' (1998b). The cornerstones of health policy are identified as:

(a) action to ensure reductions in the gaps in health status between countries and between population groups within countries;
(b) actions designed to add life to years by helping people to achieve, and use, their full physical, mental and social potential;
(c) actions designed to add health to life by reducing disease and disability; and
(d) actions which add years to life by increasing life expectancy (WHO, 1998b: 2).

These foundations embrace an extraordinarily diverse range of public policy concerns. And the publications and statements of the European Commission, which refer to the WHO Regional Office for Europe as a valued partner and close collaborator in its public health work, have made the importance EU/WHO collaboration crystal clear (CEC, 1997b: 103, 106; EU: Article 152, Para. 3).

A broader role in health – and a limited one

When discussing and reviewing amendments proposed to the key EU Public Health Treaty Article (Article 129) Ken Collins MEP (Chair of the European Parliament Committee for the Environment, Public Health and Consumer Protection, CEPHCP) observed that: '. . . the new draft treaty commits the EU to a much broader approach which now corresponds more closely with the ethos of other organisations such as the WHO' (1998b: 1). The sub-headings to be found in the Public Health chapter of the WHO Regional Report on *Health in Europe 1997* makes quite explicit what concern with health and health-related policies in Europe means and how great a range of policy areas it embraces:

- healthy lifestyles
- policies to encourage non-smoking
- sensible drinking
- psychoactive drugs: related deaths and crime in Europe
- healthy nutrition
- physical activity

- controlling risk factors related to lifestyle
- healthy public policy
- a healthy environment
- data indicators (and health)
- from planning to action (environment and health)
- safe drinking water
- air quality
- foodborne diseases
- waste management
- health promotion at work
- appropriate health care
- health care systems balancing solidarity and competition
- health care reform – policies and process
- managing change – the roles of the state, the market and centralized health systems
- primary health care (strengthening)
- hospital care
- the quest to improve the quality of care (WHO, 1998b: 45–75).

Article 129 of the Treaty on European Union (TEU) appears to be consistent with an all encompassing view of health and public policy. Asserting, as it does, that: 'Health protection requirements shall form a constituent part of the Community's other policies.' The Article, following revision at Amsterdam in October 1997, now defines the Union's responsibilities for health even more broadly and strongly: 'A high level of human health protection shall be ensured in the definition and implementation of all Community policies and activities' (EC, 1997: 108).

Like so much else that has to do with the European project the public health Article is open to rival interpretations. But, even allowing for differences of interpretation, its scope is impressive. Integrating health policy and health-related concerns into every aspect of the work of the European Commission is an awesome responsibility. Dr William Hunter, commenting on the obligations established by Article 129, in his capacity as Director of the Public Health Unit of the European Commission, wrote that there was a 'complex interaction between policy fields when it comes to health issues'. Taking as an example drugs policy he noted that:

> drugs policy constitutes a field of action within public health, as well as in the context of justice and home affairs and external relations. In addition, drugs-related projects are being funded in the context of

social policy and the Youth for Europe programme. . . . Health protection requirements have to be taken into account early on in policy development, and care should be taken that they are retained and strengthened in the decision making process. All Community Institutions are responsible for this'.

(1996: 4–5)

Of course, the European Commission has to walk a tightrope. It must not interfere directly in the health service provisions and policies of member states. It must be careful to avoid embarrassing the member states it has been created to serve. The Union Treaty states that: 'Community action in the field of public health shall fully respect the responsibilities of member states for the organisation and delivery of health services and medical care' (EC, 1997: 109). This statement of the principle of subsidiarity in relation to health seems to leave little room for misunderstanding. But the political and practical problems of managing European health policy-making, within the constraints set by this clause, are not hard to imagine. Jacques Bury, the Executive Director of the Association of Schools of Public Health in the European Region (ASPHER) complained – in *Eurohealth* in Autumn 1998 – that member state governments had opposed measures to promote harmonisation of health care services. He criticised political leaders who were not prepared to confront the frustrations – which he felt were certain to grow – among the European public who expected Europe's leaders to do more to generalise the best standards of European medicine and health care. The real problem – he suggested – was an unrealistic and obstructive attitude to the interpretation of the public health Treaty obligations. When commenting on the proposed text for the amended Article on the public health responsibilities of the EU and its Commission, in the summer of 1997, Padraig Flynn, the European Commissioner with responsibility for public health, seemed to share this view. He confessed that he had been disappointed by changes in the TEU that had confined the role of the EC to simply proposing harmonisation measures. He complained that an amendment was needed which would 'provide the Commission with an adequate legal basis to address future concerns'. He went on to explain that he feared that 'we will be confronted with a new public health threat without the means to react at Community level' (Belcher, 1997a: 2).

The European experience with Bovine Spongiform Encephalopathy (BSE) has conditioned Europe's political leaders to think in terms of great threats to public health. It has not, as yet, brought them to a point where they are prepared to do more than contemplate an enhanced role – for the European Commission and the EP – in what have traditionally been regarded as purely domestic health care issues. The balancing skills required – at the Commission and elsewhere – to stay on the tightrope above the domestic health-policy arenas of member states, while advancing the cause of European public health, need to be exemplary.

EC/EU health and health-related roles and responsibilities

Aside from specific public health activities, which the European Commission is expected to manage, it has a major role in determining the conditions under which new pharmaceuticals are released into European health-care markets. The Commission also has an important role in facilitating the free movement of medically qualified personnel and of other health professionals. And it is important, in listing the roles and responsibilities that fall to the EU, not to overlook the longest standing health-related activity for which EC institutions have been responsible – the promotion of safety and health at work.

Even if the EU had decided, as a matter of principle, to steer clear of health it would have found it impossible to do so. Jencks and Schieber – when posing questions about the containment of health-care costs – make the point that contemporary health care systems are vastly important economic enterprises. Viewed in terms of the numbers of people employed and the financial resources invested in them health care systems have become the first world's leading employers – the world's largest single industry (Jencks and Schieber, 1991). The cost and economic importance of health care systems, as well as their significance as purchasers of goods and services, means that apart from any of its public health responsibilities the EU would inevitably find itself – in fulfilling its responsibilities under the Single European Act (SEA) (the legislation that created the (SEM) in Europe) – deeply involved in health care.

Given its regulatory role the European Commission cannot escape a deep involvement in the European markets in which goods and services, as well as the services of health-service staff, are bought and sold. Supplying health care systems with medical devices – as well as pharmaceuticals – and a wide range of other goods and services is very big business. It is becoming bigger business. It is becoming more economically significant as the pace of research and development accelerates and feeds through to, often very expensive, medical innovations and developments. Innovations which are intended to capture markets outside of the EU – not just within it. The economic success of major health service suppliers is a vital element in the Union's success in international markets – something that the European Commission would be ill advised to ignore and is unlikely to ignore, when deciding how to regulate European markets supplying European health-care systems. Clinical practice and health care systems have been relatively slow to adapt to and embrace an avalanche of innovations in computing and information systems. Health services have to process and record vast amounts of information – much of it personal information. Here again the EU cannot fail to become involved in issues that are important for health-care systems and users of health services, even though it is required to keep clear of direct involvement in member state health care systems.

But the EU is much more than a free trade area – a single market. It is a community of law. The laws that underpin the single market and ultimately enforce treaty obligations in the EU are upheld and interpreted by the European Court of Justice (ECJ). The ECJ, not to be confused with the European Court of Human Rights, is the EU's supreme court. Its authority is based on the acceptance, by member states, that Community law is paramount. The role of the ECJ in European social policy has developed strongly in recent years and is growing in significance for health and health-related European policy. Specialists in European Law, Ruth Nielsen and Erica Szyszczak, have claimed that the 'ECJ has played a pivotal role in elevating certain social rights – notably in the area of free movement of persons and equal treatment between men and women into fundamental rights in EU law, protected by the ECJ and binding upon member states'. As they make clear 'the development of general principles of EU law, for example, proportionality, equality, non-discrimination have played an important role in firming up skeletal social policy provisions' (1997: 55). The ECJ is likely to be called upon to decide many critical health and health-related questions in the 21st Century and current European health policy-makers, as well as would be European health policy-makers, would do well to bear that in mind.

Commerce, science and medicine make a potent mixture in which the law frequently becomes involved. It seems highly likely that a variety of issues, connected with the human genome project, the genetic modification of food and advances in reproductive science, will eventually have to be decided at the level of the ECJ. It will be interesting to see to what extent the general principles of EU law shape laws throughout the EU on medicines, food technologies and the application of genetic research to human reproduction. It will also be interesting to observe the extent to which EU legislation and policy act as an engine, for the process of elaborating EU law on health and health-related matters and lead to a convergence of health policy in member states. An account in the *New Scientist* of the interaction of culture, politics, commerce, genetics and law, which led the Icelandic Parliament to consider licensing *deCode Genetics*, a private company in Reykjavík 'funded mainly by American investors, to manage . . . a database containing genetic, genealogical and medical details about all Icelanders', provides a flavour of the kinds of issues which are likely to find their way to the ECJ in the future (Coghlan, 1998).

Subsidiarity – a blessing in disguise?

The range of policy concerns and the cocktail of issues described above – suggesting as it does a great role for the EU and its Commission in health and health-related policy-making – needs to be tempered and qualified. The theoretical reach of the EU and its institutions greatly exceeds their grasp. There are and there will remain very substantial breaks on the EU's role in health-care and health-related policy-making. The principal formal break has already been mentioned. It is contained in the TEU – it is the subsidiarity clause (EC, 1997: Article 5, 44; Petersen, 1999: 57) and it is specifically built into Article 152 of the consolidated European Treaties. EU institutions must '. . . fully respect the responsibilities of the member states for the organisation and delivery of health services and medical care' (EC, 1997: 109). At every point in Title XII of the TEU, the Public Health title, it is made clear that Community action should depend on gaining the trust and winning the firm support of member states – the Commission is not a free agent. Community action is required to: 'complement' the activities of member states, 'promote co-ordination', 'encourage co-operation', 'foster co-operation' and 'lend support'. Only 'in close contact with member states' may the Commission 'take any useful initiative'. The legal limitations on policy-formulation, development and implementation, which are made explicit in the TEU, will generate conflict and affect the pace at which EU health and health-related policies can be developed and implemented. But the limits on the competence of the European Commission – particularly the application of the principal of subsidiarity – may be a blessing in disguise for European institutions and the Commission. That is, if the Commission and other key EU institutions are motivated – above all else – by a desire to advance the cause of public health.

Shaping a European health-care system is a very different business from shaping and reshaping national health services. Despite what Rob Baggott (1998) has called the 'revival of public health', in his study of British health care and the NHS, changing the balance of activities in national health care systems is an immensely difficult task because of 'the power of vested interests'. Those vested interests are present and well represented in the deliberations of EU institutions but they are not quite as close to the heart of the Commission's health-policy making process as they are to the core of health-care systems like the NHS. As Baggott puts it: '. . . the dominant professional interests (in Britain's health care system) are closely tied to care and treatment services and are likely to oppose radical moves to shift resources towards prevention' (1998: 295). Though they may be few in number, the officials and professionals and those European Parliamentarians, who are most interested in health-policy issues, are in a much stronger position to stand aside from the business of managing health services and to focus on the development of health policy in its broadest sense. The requirement, built into the TEU, for distance from national health-care delivery systems can also be read as detachment from the clamour for bigger and bigger investments in treatment services. Those who live their political and administrative lives in the glare of public criticism, targeted on service inadequacies and unmet needs, may come to value the encouragement and support of health-policy-makers who can see the bigger picture and offer them a European and continent-wide perspective on how best to serve the public interest. This book is, at least in part, an attempt to capture and reflect that continental supranational perspective on health policy.

It is, of course, important to constantly bear in mind the modesty of the resources that the Commission has available. In his forward to *Public Health in Europe* (CEC, 1997b), Padraig Flynn, refers to the 'mounting demands being made' upon the resources of Union member states to 'meet the pressures of rapidly changing medical technology, ageing populations and ever growing needs for health care and social support'. These factors were held to explain the average 7.4 per cent share of member states Gross Domestic Product (GDP) being devoted to health care (CEC, 1997b: 5, 9). It is worth contrasting this level of spending by member state health care systems with the amount invested in the European Commission's work on health and health-related issues.

The Commission has very limited financial and human resources to make its contribution to health policy. Andrew Hayes, President of the European Public Health Alliance, wrote in 1998, that: '. . . the European Commission employs fewer people than a large county council in England' (1998: 2). Only a small fraction of European Commission staff are committed to work on health issues. Indeed the Commission's resources for work on health issues have been compared unfavourably with those available to the British Health Education Authority, a national health organisation which is devoted exclusively to health promotion and education work in just one member state (Randall, 1997: 293).

Ali El-Agraa, in one of the standard works on the EU, has compared the EU's total budget in 1997 with the resources available to 'a large UK (government) department'. A cap was imposed on EU expenditure in 1992 – this limited its rate of growth and set a ceiling of 1.27 per cent of EU GDP on EU spending in 1999. Only about 5 per cent of the EU budget total is spent on administration and the cost of *eurocrats* and EU interpreters and translators is frequently exaggerated (El-Agraa, 1998: 318–19). As is well known, most EU spending goes on supporting farm prices, the Common Agricultural Policy (CAP). The CAP accounted for around 55 per cent of the total budget in the early 1990s and was projected to fall to 46 per cent by the end of the century (Nugent, 1994: 344). So-called structural operations represent around one-third of EU spending and these resources have to be shared out between the European Regional Development Fund (ERDF) and the European Social Fund (ESF). The resources available for specific public health initiatives and programmes are a tiny proportion of the EU budget and likely to remain so. This is for two very obvious reasons: the scale of EU spending on agricultural price support and the strength of competition for EU funds from other quarters within the EU.

Readers can get some idea of the modesty of public health-programme spending from the published figures for EU spending on its biggest, best known and longest established public health programme, *Europe Against Cancer*. The third plan to fight cancer, which built on a programme initiated in 1986, was designed to last five years (1996–2000). It was allocated Ecu-64 million (DGV, 1998a: 2). The European currency unit (Ecu) was replaced by the common European currency (Euro) on a 1:1 basis on 1 January 1999. The Euro was worth approximately two-thirds of the pound sterling – shortly after its adoption at the beginning of 1999. So the third *Europe Against Cancer* plan was being supported by the annual sterling equivalent of around £8.5 million. The plan – along with other public health initiatives managed directly by the Commission – will be the focus of a chapter devoted to EU public-health programmes later in this book.

With so great a canvas on which to paint and limited by the terms of the TEU and the resources available to them the supporters of the new public health and the officials and professionals working on health and health-related issues in the Commission need powerful allies. Without those allies they will find it very difficult to play a constructive part in ensuring that a high level of human health protection is built into 'the definition and implementation of all Community policies and activities'.

Members of the Euro-health lobby have shown little hesitation in identifying the European public as their most powerful potential ally.

Carol Ludvigsen and Kathleen Roberts, in their *Health Care Policies in Europe – implications for practice*, issue a clarion call to the European public and to their fellow health-care professionals, to get serious about the EU and its role in health (1996: 1–3). It will be necessary, however, if European public opinion is to be brought to bear on European health-policy making, to connect what EU institutions do much more strongly with subjects that arouse and mobilise the public. The Europe wide concern about BSE has shown that there are issues capable of mobilising something that might reasonably be described as European public opinion. But unleashing European public opinion may not, if the warnings of Petersen and Lupton are taken seriously, be all plain sailing; irrationality, prejudice and authoritarianism can feed off public fears about strangers and the often ill-defined risks associated with scientific and technological innovation (1996: 174–81). An informed and rational debate about highly emotive subjects like food safety is hard to create and even harder to sustain, even among those who share a common political culture and have a clear understanding of the institutions through which policy (European and national) is formulated and implemented.

The challenge of making Europe count with its public

The strongest proponents of a radical role for the EU, when advancing the cause of the new public health and much else besides, generally make it clear that they are aware that it is necessary to make the institutions of the EU more potent and more democratic (Townsend, 1992a). They acknowledge that this is unlikely to happen without more public involvement and commitment to Europe and its political institutions. They also acknowledge that the relationship between the European public and Europe's political institutions is rather like the relationship between the chicken and the egg. You cannot have one without the other and both, when challenged about their inability to take the lead, explain that the other comes first. The future of European health policy is – in the eyes of Euro-health lobbyists – twinned, however unhappily, with the advance of EU democracy.

Andrew Hayes, in his role as President of the European Public Health Alliance (EPHA), writing in 1998 about the EU and public health beyond the year 2000, found some grounds to be hopeful about engaging the interest of 'fickle' EU citizens in European health-policy-making. 'For a few short months', in response to cross-border health risks – Acquired Immune Deficiency Syndrom (AIDS) and BSE/Creutzfeldt-Jakob Disease (CJD), 'MEPs reversed their normal sense of political priorities' – health went from 'near the bottom to the top of the pile'. To sustain and build on this interest Hayes insists that it is up to the EU's political leaders, on the basis of a 'rigorous, comprehensive, and evidence-based . . . approach to policy analysis' – clearly the responsibility of the public health professionals – to demonstrate leadership and convince EU citizens that 'a self-assured, vibrant and responsive Europe is good for our health' (1998: 2–4). Such a view runs straight into the studied and considered scepticism of political scientists and policy analysts such as Stephan Leibfried and Paul Pierson (1995), who believe that the EU is more likely than not to be let down by its political institutions.

Recognising that historically federal institutions are planned and constructed to ration the amount of political authority concentrated at any one point Pierson and Leibfried remark that: 'Multitiered institutional settings . . . serve to fragment political authority (and thereby) create dilemmas for policymakers.' How is it possible to share power and get anything done? Pierson and Leibfried review, at some length, the formidable obstacles to EU policy-making and the pressures to adopt lowest-common-denominator strategies, recommendations and 'solutions'. Does the EU – because its policy-making machinery and political institutions are complex and reliant on the co-operation of a very large number of players – face a gridlocked future? Hope of a politically productive future, in the social policy area, rests – so far as Leibfried and Pierson are concerned – on two factors. The necessity – if member states want to preserve and protect the single market they have created – for the member states to respect the paramount role of the ECJ and the relative absence of impediments to decision-making by the ECJ itself. Secondly, the acceptance of qualified majority voting (QMV) for reaching agreement on a greater range of social issues (Liebfried and Pierson, 1995: 457–65). The Public Health article, Article 152 of the consolidated Treaty on EU, contains the following words: 'The Council, acting by a qualified majority on a proposal from the Commission, may also adopt recommendations for the purposes set out in this article.'

From the point of view of Andrew Hayes – and others, who share his enthusiasm for a bolder and more determined EU role in health-policy-making – Liebfried and Pierson do have a few encouraging words. Encouragement that extends to the writer of this book. Liebfried and Pierson argue that: 'The European Union is a polity in the making. A great deal is up for grabs' (1995: 464). The widening, deepening and strengthening of the European polity will surely depend upon the relevance of European policy-making, in health as in many other areas, to the lives of Europe's citizens and the competition for votes among the

EU's national and supranational politicians. The means by which European citizens and health professionals, who are interested in the EU's health policies, can exert influence on them through the EU's institutions, its lobby groups and in other ways, is clearly an important subject for this book. One essential requirement is a better understanding of the policies themselves.

The structure of the book and the topics covered

As the chapter headings and organisation of this book indicate, the linkages between the lives of European citizens and the health and health-related policy-making activities of the EU are numerous and diverse. In this penultimate section of the introductory chapter the structure of the book will be presented and explained. My aim is to communicate the EU's considerable reach and involvement in health and health-related questions as well as the intensely political character of many of the most important health-policy issues with which the EU is concerned. The book begins with a discussion and investigation of the Community's role in health and safety at work. It is the longest established health/health-related, responsibility of the EC. Nation states, which agree to open up their markets to one another – and endorse the principles of free trade among themselves – have good reason to be concerned about the rules that affect the trading game. There is good reason for all concerned to make it clear that their support for and willingness to go along with free trade is conditional upon it also being fair.

Whatever intrinsic value effective health and safety legislation has – and improving the working conditions of all of Europe's workers was integral to Monnet's vision of Europe – it is quite fundamental as a means of controlling, and ultimately outlawing, commercial strategies that rely upon employers and producers neglecting risks to the health and well-being of their workers and the public at large. Health and safety legislation is not simply about making the working environment safe it is about preventing *social dumping*. Social dumping can be defined as leaving others to make provision for and bear the costs and consequences of dangerous and unhealthy working environments. The costs of a dangerous or unhealthy working environment are left to fall where they may, most often on workers and their families.

Competitive advantages gained by neglecting the interests of employees have been a particular focus of EC activities. The EC's directives and policy-making in this area offers rich illustration of the theme of spill over in EU policy. And the linkages between trade and competition policy and multifarious other policy issues – including health-policy issues – for which the EU has responsibility. Chapter 3, dealing with the relationship between the health professions and the EU, concentrates on the implications and implementation of one of the EC's core objectives – unfettered movement for Community citizens. The right to live and work in any member state, which the Treaty of Rome enshrines, has proven far from easy to implement. The mutual recognition of professional qualifications by member states and the harmonisation of training schemes, that such mutual recognition necessitates, has been a severe test for the EC and has – on more than one occasion – required a radical rethink by the European Commission, in approach and methodology. The complexity and size of health-service labour markets in Europe and suspicions about the quality of training of medical practitioners – qualifying in different member states – has meant that EU policies, directives and decisions, about qualifications, have the potential to affect professional mobility and thus have ramifications for health-care systems throughout the EU.

There is little doubt that European idealists look to the members of the leading professions – such as medicine, which includes some of Europe's best-educated citizens – to blaze a trail towards a EU in which national identity matters less and enlightenment values, belief in rationality and tolerance of cultural diversity, matter far more. Genuine freedom of movement for professionals – as well as for all other workers – is an important part of the European project proposed by Monnet. The book's fourth chapter is concerned with one of the success stories of the 20th Century; an industry that supplies health-care systems around the world and which produces and promises to go on producing some of the highest levels of profitability for the owners of capital in the world, the pharmaceutical industry. The Treaty of Rome – the foundation of the EEC free market, as modified by the SEA – was designed to create a market for pharmaceutical manufacturers in which unjustified constraints on the trade in pharmaceuticals were swept away. The determination to remove barriers to free trade in medicines came into conflict with the desire of member states to protect their domestic pharmaceutical industry and to safeguard the public health by maintaining national controls on the testing and introduction of new medicines.

The EU now has a medicines evaluation agency (the European Agency for the Evaluation of Medicinal Products (EMEA), based in London. It has the task of ensuring that common standards apply to all new medicines – so that there can be something more like a single market in new medicines. Of course, harmonisation of the procedures for introducing new drugs leads on to other things; to what extent should the EU or an EU agency concern itself with the efficacy of drugs, their cost or the ways in which they are sold? These are issues that are both intensely commercial and political at the same time. The pharmaceutical industry itself is increasingly organised in firms that have a global reach – not simply a European one. The relationship between companies that represent themselves as great innovators, working on behalf of humankind (as well as a most successful branch of European capitalism), and an EU which is obliged to look after the interests of the European public at the same time as it polices free trade, make the relationship between the Union and the pharmaceutical industry an especially fascinating study.

Chapter 5, the final chapter in Part I, is concerned with the rise of the EU's public-health competence. Although the sums of money available to the European Commission, as has already been illustrated, are modest it is obvious that there is a great sense of pride in the Commission about what its public-health programmes have achieved and about what they represent in terms of defining common concerns and a common purpose in European public-health policy-making. In the final edition of its publication *Prevention*, for 1997, the Director of the European Commission's Public Health Unit, Dr W.J. Hunter, identified a list of eight programmes that the European Commission had developed or was developing to address priority diseases and health issues. He wrote:

> The diseases for which specific programmes have either been adopted or proposed include cancer, AIDS and other communicable diseases, drug dependence, pollution related diseases, accidents and injuries, as well as rare diseases. In addition two more general programmes on health promotion, information, education and training and on health monitoring have been adopted . . .
>
> (DGV, 1997b: 1)

The Director went on to assert his strong belief in the role that the EC could play, should '. . . member states agree to improve collaboration on health care matters' (DGV, 1997b: 1). The first six programmes referred to will be considered in detail in the fifth chapter – more general programmes and concerns will be considered in Part II of the book.

Part II of this book looks to the future and at the recent past. Part II begins with Chapter 6 entitled, 'BSE, Health and Risk in the EU'. It focuses on the impact that BSE and the new variant of Creutzfeldt-Jakob Disease (nvCJD) has had on European health and health-related policy-making. BSE has scared people across Europe and provoked and empowered EU institutions to intervene in a member state's affairs in a quite extraordinary and unparalleled fashion in order to deal with concern about 'mad cows' and the threat to the health of the humans that they represent. nvCJD is, however, just one of a number of health scares and crises which, to use the words of David Davis, underline the fact that contemporary western 'democracies are . . . [highly] risk averse' (Bate, 1999: vii). The risks which may stoke fires of EC concern and harness public opinion to identify and support action on common interests, from one side of the world's largest single market to the other, may also impel EU policy-makers to decisions that are short-sighted, ill-informed, and ineffective. That are, not to put too fine a point on it, panicky and narrowly party political (Everest, 1999: 242–58). The risks and threats to the public health, which are often presented to the public as a cocktail of science, politics and inflammatory reporting, seem to be ubiquitous. On the other hand the potential of medical science and medical technologies seem boundless, almost miraculous; even if we are far from certain about the motives and trustworthiness of many of those who market them.

How is an EU, which is said to rest on four pillars – free movement of people, of goods and services and of capital – to find a way of combining commercial freedom and prosperity with respect for individuals, their interests, wishes and priorities? Some have suggested that politics is largely irrelevant, markets will nearly always do a better job that the political process. It is best to leave markets alone to allocate scarce resources as efficiently as possible. Markets will provide as good a resolution of differences as is possible by any other means. There are many who believe that the flaws in political institutions – quite aside from the flaws evident in individual politicians – make them highly ineffective instruments for steering a course for society. It is possible that, even with the very best of intentions, the knowledge, will and capacity to make informed policy decisions democratically is lacking.

However, Europe can claim to be the world's most diverse, developed and sophisticated polity. It is a test case for international co-operation and governance. Whether it is led principally by elected politicians or by lawyers, Commissioners or expert public servants, the EU appears rather better placed to serve, as an international pilot, than any other supranational form of government currently available. EU politics and European political institutions provide us with a test case; how far is it possible for economic competitors to work successfully together to protect and improve the public health?

As the treaty obligation to ensure that a high level of human health protection is now a part of all EC/EU policies and activities any serious attempt to give the commitment expression will depend on knowledge-able and capable policy-makers. If they are to be effective they must be able to convince, regulate or frighten others into accepting that there is a bigger picture that can be comprehended and acted upon. Democrats will no doubt hope that such policy-makers are willing and able to explain themselves to others and to seek popular support for the policies that they recommend.

The complexity and difficulty of forming judgements about potential health risks and conveying them, in a balanced way, to others makes the task of finding and retaining effective policy-makers and advisers a very difficult one. Many of those who are best qualified and have most to offer to the EU and to member states will no doubt also have offers of employment in organisations which have substantial pecuniary interests in shaping EU health and health-related policy.

Chapter 7 deals with the work that the EU and – most especially – its Commission is expected to undertake to encourage, promote and assist member states to: 'make their health systems as effective as possible' (CEC, 1997b: 5). In 1991 the Health Ministers of EU member states adopted a resolution on 'fundamental health choices'. Padraig Flynn explains, in his foreword to *Choices in Health Policy: An Agenda for the European Union* (Abel-Smith, 1995a), that the Commission called on Professor Brian Abel-Smith and his academic colleagues to write a report on 'the organization of health services and the issues that member states have to address in framing their policies for the future' (xi). Although the European Commission is prohibited from itself becoming directly involved in the delivery of medical care in member states it clearly sees a role for the EU in facilitating the exchange of ideas and information about the difficult choices facing contemporary health-care systems.

Chapter 7 also considers the application of telematics in health-care and health-care systems. It has to be acknowledged that telematics is a rather off-putting term. According to the technical directory, which readers can consult by visiting the the European Telematics Horizontal Observatory Service (ETHOS – which forms part of the EU's Telematics Application Programme), the term telematics is: 'derived from the French word "Telematique" and refers to the use of computers alongside telecommu-nications systems . . . [T]elematics ranges from all forms of dial-up service, through the Internet, and on to broadband applications such as Full Service Network'.

Through its Health Care Sector Strategic Requirements Board, the European Commission has sought in recent years to determine how the EU's fifth framework programme could 'serve to speed up the ongoing building of Community based, distributed healthcare IT infrastructure in the member states and help to make this activity a European industrial activity with a global scope' (CEC, 1998b). In its, Report on the Telematics Applications Programme, the Board, Chaired by Jean-Claude Healy, begins by observing that: 'European healthcare is . . . undergoing . . . a paradigm . . . shift from healthcare institution-centred care to a citizen-centred care'; it is a shift which, readers are told, 'implies a decentralised health care where services, with evidence based effectiveness, are available to all and are provided in a way (which makes) . . . organisational boundaries . . . invisible to the citizen'. Healy and his colleagues are clear: 'Information and communication technologies (ICT) . . . (will come increasingly to support and improve) health services by providing . . . direct access to specialised national or European health and medical knowledge' (Healy, 1997: 4–7).

The European Commission is seeking to place itself in the vanguard of the application of the information revolution in health-care across the EU. Clearly it has neither the financial nor the human resources to do more than signpost and encourage the application of ICT to Europe's health-care systems, but the ambition and scope of the role it is seeking to carve out for itself would undoubtedly excite and enthuse Jean Monnet. Nevertheless it is appropriate to ask to what extent the development of telematics can be expected to enable Europeans to learn from each other and to make their health-care systems more effective? How far and how quickly will member states and their citizens be able to follow this particular pied piper? A key and highly instrumental role in the facilitating the distribution of high-quality health-care information, in support of effective health services, among vast numbers of people over great distances at relative low cost is, understandably, a prospect which greatly excites the European Commission.

In 1994, Margaret Whitehead, the author of *The Health Divide*, a report on health inequalities, which was most unwelcome to the British Government of the day, wrote an Editorial for the *European Journal of Public Health*; her article was entitled 'Why not now?: action on inequalities in health' (Whitehead and Dahlgren, 1994: 1–2; see also Townsend, 1992: 6–9). The Editorial sought to emphasise the relationship between what is now widely labelled *social exclusion* and poor health. In doing so it also sought to underline the importance – for health policy-makers – of social and economic policy measures designed to reduce material inequalities. Chapter 8 of this book focuses on what is undoubtedly the most testing and politically explosive health-policy issue for the EU: its willingness and capacity to design and implement measures which redistribute wealth and income among EU citizens. Carles Muntaner and John Lynch (1999) describe the work of the social epidemiologist, Richard Wilkinson, on social inequality and health status, as the 'leading research programme in social epidemiology'; Wilkinson has demonstrated that 'population health is strongly associated with the distribution of income' (1996: 59, 61).

The principal implication of the Wilkinson research programme, for social epidemiology and health-policy-making, is that policies which increase disposable income, while preserving or increasing income differentials, will fail to reduce inequalities in health. Redistribution from rich to poor is presented as potentially critical – perhaps even decisive – in improving the health of millions of Europe's poorer citizens. The considerable differences in health status, which Abel-Smith and his colleagues reported – between member states, social classes, occupational groups, regions, men and women and ethnic groups – provide plenty of justification for 'policy-relevant research' and for European social policies, aimed at combating social exclusion. Indeed the report urged the 'Community . . . [to] . . . press ahead with its initiative to establish a minimum income for each member state as evidence [accumulates] that inadequate income is itself health-damaging' (Abel-Smith *et al.*, 1995: 139–40).

The concluding chapter identifies and reviews the major themes of the book. A press release issued by the Commission in July 1997 described the Union's *Agenda 2000* as a plan 'for a stronger and wider Europe' (Commission PR, 1997a: 3–16). It claimed that *Agenda 2000* represented a 'comprehensive response' to requests received from the European Council, which met in Madrid in December 1995, to map out the future of the EU and to take the EU beyond the year 2000. The Union was faced with 'an historic turning point for Europe', it would be substantially enlarged and it would need to be equipped to meet the challenges of a rapidly changing international and domestic environment. That meant that it would need to reform its institutions, so that they were sufficiently adaptable to respond successfully to 'certain *long-term trends*' (emphasis added). The long-term trends referred to included: 'the concerns of the man and woman in the street, population trends, new technologies, restructuring of markets and enterprises, and the globalisation of the economy and the emergence of a multi-polar world'. The release even went so far as to describe the *Agenda 2000* Union priority goal as *economic and social cohesion*, asserting that: 'the prospect of enlargement encompassing new countries with widely diverging levels of development makes this even more necessary than before'.

If we believe that good health is something that has value beyond measure, or even if we take a more worldly view – that it has great value, while not quite being ineffable or immeasurable – *Agenda 2000* invites us all to judge the EU by its successes and failures in promoting social cohesion. Protecting and improving the health of Europe's citizens is a matter of no little importance then. Of course the aims we associate with health and health-related policies often come into conflict and health is not all that citizens and their elected representatives care about. Building healthier societies – as the discussion contained in the final chapter of the book seeks to affirm – will remain an intensely political and fascinating part of the EU story.

War and peace

It would be inappropriate, in a book that is about European politics, as well as European health-policy, not to make a final point, in concluding the introduction to the book. Europeans should never lose sight of one of the greatest contributions to health made by the EU and the EC upon which it has been built – the contribution that integrating supranational institutions and laws make to maintaining the peace. The absence of such integrating institutions and of the common commercial life that has grown up over fifty years in Western Europe is all too apparent in Asia and other parts of Europe. Whatever local difficulties exist and have existed in the Balkans, it is in Asia that international, not just regional, peace is threatened by the lack of institutions to create and sustain the international equivalent of neighbourliness. The suspicion, hostility and distrust that exists between India and Pakistan and the want of institutions strong enough to forge closer and deeper relation between India and China must be counted among the greatest of contemporary threats to the longevity and well-being of millions of human beings. As long as the EU prospers and member states remain at peace with one another Monnet's Europe, of common rules and institutions, will be making a very considerable contribution to the health and well-being of all its citizens.

2
Health and Safety at Work

Health and safety – part of the core

Promoting safety at work and protecting and improving the health of workers appear among the fundamental objectives for which the EC, including the first of the Communities, the ECSC, were established. Article 3e Title 1 of the ECSC Treaty called upon its signatories to 'promote improved working conditions and an improved standard of living for the workers'. Improvement of working and living conditions was to go hand in hand with the harmonisation of measures to protect and promote health in the work place. The Treaty of Rome, which established the EEC, incorporated the aims of Article 3e (see Article 117 in Gold, 1993: 214). And it gave the European Commission, under Article 118, the task of 'promoting close co-operation between member states in the social field'. Health and safety at work featured prominently among the social issues listed in the Article. Labour law and working conditions, the prevention of occupational accidents and diseases and occupational hygiene were specifically identified as matters for Commission action. The European Commission was required to make studies, deliver opinions and arrange consultations (Gold, 1993: 214–15; European Communities, 1997a: 101–4). As Article 118 made plain, partnership with the social partners (unions and employers) and international organisations, not just member state governments, was to be a part of the recipe for the Commission to facilitate progress in the social field.

Article 2b of the EURATOM, also signed in Rome in 1957, went further still. It linked the desire to protect the health of workers with the health of citizens in general, calling upon member states to 'establish uniform safety standards to protect the health of workers *and of the general public and ensure that they are applied*' (emphasis added). The EEC partners, also the signatories to EURATOM, agreed – as part of the provisions for implementing EURATOM – that the Council and the European Commission would be assisted in establishing and applying uniform safety standards by an Economic and Social Committee (ESC) – acting in an advisory capacity. It does not seem unreasonable to suggest that the *Monnet method* (Wallace and Wallace, 1996: 42–5, 46, 47) was once again being applied. Success in associating modest steps, with a purpose transcending national interests but not inconsistent with them, might provide just the encouragement needed by would be co-operators to build and consolidate collaboration between Europe's constituent nations.

EURATOM – a model for action

However, fine sounding words about protecting the interests of workers would never be enough for true co-operators. There was little of real substance in most of the ECSC, EURATOM and EEC Treaty provisions targeted at improving health and safety at work. The lack of substance led Phil James, in his review of the origins of European health and safety measures, to describe the key Treaty articles as 'statements of intent' which were not 'backed up by any specific legislative powers'. James does, nevertheless, record a notable exception (James, 1993: 136). The exception was Community action to regulate materials that produced ionising radiation.

Nuclear materials were thought to require special scientific under-standing and special measures. They were linked with serious potential – but ill-defined – hazards. Most political leaders, along with the general public, found it hard to be sure about what was at stake and to confidently assess the dangers. The new Community, EURATOM, was established to deal with something that seemed to be full of economic and scientific promise, but which was also easy to represent as a very serious threat to public health.

Chapter 3 of the EURATOM Treaty was intended to put in place a common machinery to deal with the threat that nuclear technology represented, without obstructing scientific and economic progress. A search for an accommodation between economic and safety considerations – something that is at the core of occupational health and safety policy-making – was initiated. Indeed the EURATOM Treaty provisions can be read as a model for a process which has become increasingly familiar in the EC/EU; with the formulation, agreement and then the application of standards and regulations designed to protect people in the workplace – and beyond – from risky processes, activities and materials. Articles 30–39 of the EURATOM Treaty required the members of the European Atomic Energy Community (EAEC) to:

1. *Lay down basic and enforceable standards* to protect the health of workers and the general public against dangers arising from ionising radiation.
2. *Empower the Commission to draw up recommendations* about basic standards, through a detailed consultative process, and forward proposals to EC institutions for agreement (subject to qualified majority voting) prior to implementation throughout Community member states.
3. *Develop a dynamic process for setting standards*, one capable of being developed in the light of new scientific information and the experience of individual member states.
4. *Develop arrangements to ensure that member states comply with and enforce basic standards* – allowing for different national methodologies to be used in doing so.
5. Make use of EC institutions and resources to *establish ways and means to educate and train* all those who need to be informed and equipped to deal with hazards.
6. *Work through the Commission to harmonise specific measures* needed to deal with hazards.
7. *Set timetables for formulating and presenting new plans and proposals* for action.
8. *Make use of the Commission to share information about particular risks* and to deal with hazards which pose a threat beyond the boundaries of an individual member state;
9. *Require member states to monitor and record hazards* and to make such information available to the Commission (so that it could be shared with other member states and used to assess the efficiency with which hazards were being measured and dealt with).;
10. *Require the Commission to develop and publish an informed view of particular hazards*;
11. Allow, where there had been a breach Treaty obligations, for *compliance to be enforced through the ECJ*; and,
12. *Establish a specialist body to undertake research*, collect information and provide technical and scientific support to the Commission and inform discussion and policy making throughout the Community.

Calling on the experts and working with the grain

Of course EURATOM may be dismissed as a *very* special case. But, as is clear from the European Commission's own account of the work of the ECSC and the evolution of the EU's occupational health and safety role (DGV, 1999c), it can also be understood as entirely congruent with initiatives that preceded it: initiatives designed to reduce the risks associated with working in coal mines and other extractive industries.

The difficulties of proceeding across a broad front to promote health and safety at work were however much greater. The ECSC and EURATOM put great emphasis on involving experts. Indeed it was the ECSC that began the process of consulting: ' . . . professional organisations, governments and scientists within the framework of specific committees . . .'; addressing 'problems in relation to health protection of the workers in the coal and steel industries; the development and publication of statistics on accidents at work', and supporting systematic studies aimed at helping workers who had been injured at work. By 1957 the ECSC had established a Safety and Health Commission for mining and other extractive industries 'to prevent the occurrence of major accidents' in the sector (DGV, 1999c). The architects of the European Community (EC), not just contemporary Commission historians, had concluded that one of the principal requirements for developing a multinational agreement on health and safety, covering coal mining and steel making (and capable of extension beyond them), was the presentation of proposals strongly endorsed by expert opinion. While the ECSC had sought, for some time, to draw experts into its work to reduce accidents in the mineral-extracting industries the High Authority (forerunner to the European Commission) had also learnt how important it was to work with the grain of member state opinion; to take established economic interests into account. The example of Commission and EC action, provided by the EURATOM Treaty, illustrated what could be achieved while underlining how contingent rapid progress – in building an EC competence – would be on acting decisively when the opportunity arose. A big unanswered question ten years on from the establishment of the ECSC was how far and how quickly it would be possible to develop and generalise wide-ranging agreements on occupational health and safety.

This chapter describes and discusses the way in which the ECs have, in the course of the last 40 years, come to play an increasingly important role in health and safety at work; have been able to build on the ECSC, the Rome Treaty and draw on EURATOM, in particular, as a model for European health and safety work. In telling the story this chapter also sets out to equip the reader with an understanding of some aspects of the European policy-making process; an endeavour in which, it has to be acknowledged, it is impossible to avoid Euro jargon.

The EURATOM Treaty was concerned with risks that were associated in the public imagination with new and somewhat exotic technologies. On the other hand the ECSC and its Safety and Health Commission were concerned with raising standards and eliminating variations in occupational health and safety in industries that were much older, much more socially and economically complex and deeply integrated into member state economies. The ECSC was concerned above all else with established industries that employed very large numbers of people. From the very beginning it was clear that the ECSC put great faith in the role that expert scientific opinion could play. While clear expert scientific opinion was most unlikely, on its own, to enable the leaders of member states to find their way speedily to a comprehensive health and safety regime the Commission was (and it remains) committed to the view that expert opinion, united with enlightened self-interest, has a critical role to play. The establishment of a European Committee of Senior Labour Inspectors (SLIC) in recent years, the creation – in 1996 – of a specialist European Health and Safety Agency (EASHW) based in Spain and the earlier creation of the European Foundation for the Improvement of Living and Working Conditions (EFILWC) (based in Dublin), all continue a Commission tradition of bringing expert scientific opinion as close to the policy making process as possible (DGV, 1999c). These are all developments to which we will return.

Free trade, Fair trade and health and safety

The creation of the EEC in 1958 added another string to the High Authority/Commission's bow. It made it possible for the Commission to present proposals for improvements in occupational health and safety as a *sine qua non* for a general common market and not just a means of improving the lot of particular groups of workers. In the words of the Commission's Directorate General, charged with reviewing and developing the EU's occupational health and safety policies at the end of the 20th Century, the Treaty of Rome made '. . . the need for a global approach to health and safety of workers . . . more evident'. The Commission's greatest problem, however, was that it could not direct member states to harmonise standards, despite substantial evidence that 'there were wide differences in the measures taken on health and safety of their workers'

(DGV, 1999c). The challenge for those in the Commission, who wanted to generalise the role and powers found in the EURATOM Treaty, in relation to ionising radiation, was to win support for the idea that common standards, in regulating employment conditions, were essential and every bit as fundamental as the legal measures at the heart of the Treaty of Rome were to free trade between member states. The Commission needed to be able to do more than fund research and issue advice.

The European Commission began by issuing recommendations which it was hoped would contribute to a climate, throughout the EEC, which was favourable to harmonisation of health and safety measures. It made an Industrial Health and Safety Division, established in 1962, responsible for this work. The recommendations covered such things as arrangements for the surveillance of employees exposed to risks in the work place, occupational medicine, a European list of occupational diseases, protection of young people at work and compensation for people suffering from occupational diseases. The Safety and Health Commission for mining, set up in 1957, was given an extended role and by 1974 had become responsible for advising the European Commission about the best ways to collect and compare accident at work and health at work data. It also had responsibility for following up proposals to improve health and safety at work; suggesting research programmes into health and safety at work; facilitating the exchange of information and submitting an annual report on safety and health matters. And, following a decision of the European Council, in June 1974, an Advisory Committee for Safety, Hygiene and Health Protection at Work (ACSHH), was established. A partnership body bringing together representatives of employers, unions and governments from across the EC. The Committee went on to play a key role in drawing up the first of a series of EC action programmes on safety and health at work (which ran from 1978 to 1982). Although the Commission now claims that in the years up to 1978 it built a foundation for EC health and safety policy it describes the late 1970s and early 1980s as a period of accelerated progress. They were the years when a general European legislative foundation for occupational health and safety was laid. They were the years during which, in the Commission's terms, there was a development away 'from total dependence on national legislation towards a widespread acceptance of the role of the European Community' (DGV, 1999c). A development which the Commission claims was entirely consistent with trends in European public opinion – noting that in 1991 'a Eurobarometer survey revealed that 94 per cent of workers were in favour of common legislation for all member states' (DGV, 1999c).

Making the Rules

The Commission of the EU is charged with the responsibility for making proposals designed to benefit the EU as a whole and to further the aims of the EU. Its proposals on health and safety at work, in common with other proposals, can take a number of different forms. It can make and issue Recommendations, Regulations, Decisions and Directives. Recommendations are not binding on member states. Regulations, Decisions and Directives do have legal force. Regulations take immediate and general effect when adopted, while Decisions apply to particular parties – which may be in dispute with each other or considered by the Commission to be in breach of EC rules. Directives are binding on all member states but allow individual member states to incorporate EU provisions into their own national legislation by enacting appropriate laws.

As James puts it: 'The period from mid-1970s up to the end of 1987 . . . saw a considerable increase in EC activity in the field of occupational healthand safety, which resulted in the adoption of a number of important and significant Directives' (141–2). The Commission's ability to get its proposals for health and safety Regulations and Directives adopted was, nevertheless, inhibited by the requirement that they be agreed by all member states. Unanimity was needed before proposals could be made binding on member states. The requirement for unanimity before new Directives could be introduced was finally set aside at the end of the 1980s. The increased scope of EC legislation and the accelerating rate at which it was being adopted in the late 1980s have been attributed to a growing awareness, beginning in the 1970s, of the social and economic consequences of uneven economic growth and the introduction of QMV for some European Council decision-making (Gold, 1993: 19–21).

QMV was introduced for decisions on health and safety matters, following the passage of the SEA, in 1987. The SEA also set a date for the completion of the single market, which gave a powerful boost to the Commission's work on measures to harmonise EC rules, including health and safety measures.

The Council of Ministers has been described as the principal decision-making body within the EU (Bainbridge with Teasdale, 1995: 90). This Council (there is a European Council which is a quite distinct body) brings together representatives – elected national political leaders serving as government ministers – from member states. The Council, made up of government ministers from member states, brings those ministers together, in different combinations according to the subject matter being dealt with, to transact business across a vast range of shared European concerns. Health ministers, for example, meeting together in the Health Council, to discuss the health and health-related issues and policies of the EU. It is a process that is far from transparent. The meetings of the Council of Ministers are held behind closed doors. The introduction of QMV for health and safety matters, among others, has meant, however, that the Council, made up of representatives of the 15 EU member states, can reach a 'common position' if 62 votes – out of a possible 87 – are cast in favour of a particular proposal.

Voting power in the Council is weighted in a very approximate way to reflect population size. Four member states, France, Germany, Italy and the UK, have ten votes while Luxembourg, the smallest member state, has just two. The Council – with its ministerial make up dependent on the subjects being discussed – normally meets to deal with formal proposals presented by the European Commission. This is one of the features of the role of the Commission that makes it a very unusual supranational body. It combines 'administrative, executive, legislative and judicial activities and responsibilities' (Bainbridge with Teasdale, 1995: 160).

The EP has the power to dismiss the whole of the Commission – something that the Commission recognised when the European Commissioners, led by Jacques Santer – the Commission President in the late 1990s – resigned *en masse* in March 1999; although they did not depart until sometime later. The European Parliament has also developed an increasingly important role in policy-making, budget setting and law making – although its powers and influence are severely constrained by the greater legislative authority of the Council of Ministers (Nugent, 1994: 123–5, 174–86).

Occupational health and safety legislation is not only subject to political and policy-making processes which bring the Commission, the Council of Ministers and the EP together – and sometimes into conflict – it is also influenced by bodies which are intended to promote principles of social partnership, said to be at the core of the EC activities in the social field. Articles 138 and 139 of the Consolidated Treaty establishing the EC incorporate a commitment, which can be traced back through the history of the EC, to encourage and promote social dialogue between management and labour at European level (European Communities, 1997: 103). While, as Martin Rhodes (1995) notes, this commitment had provoked the 'hostility of capital' in the past 'by the time of Maastricht . . . employers had accepted – at least in principle – the procedural importance of rule setting at the EC level through social dialogue' (104–5). In the case of occupational health and safety measures the Advisory Committee for

Safety, Hygiene and Health Protection at Work (ACSHH) was established in order to 'assist the Commission in the preparation and implementation of activities in the field of health and safety at work . . . [and it enabled] . . . the Commission, with the agreement of both sides of industry (to initiate) a . . . co-ordinated action programme starting in 1978' (DGV, 1999c).

Apart from facilitating a scientifically and technically informed debate and making detailed proposals – which have a reasonable prospect of getting the agreement of at least a qualified majority of the Council of Ministers – the Commission has been seeking to foster agreement and co-operation between employers and workers throughout Europe. The Advisory Committee has been its principal instrument for this work for more than a quarter of a century. The Commission clearly regards the Advisory Committee's role as vital in advancing the cause of health and safety at work.

Starting to review results and achievements

What have the Commission and its partners achieved? What have the results of European health and safety action programmes and legislative proposals been? What is the EU capable of achieving? A vast number of European Directives and Regulations have been introduced. There is a framework of European law that affects many different aspects of the working environment and can be argued to provide protection in the workplace and, in a significant number of cases, beyond it. It is worth pointing out that not all of the European legislation, which is relevant to occupational health and safety, has been introduced under treaty provisions specifically concerned with the workplace. Articles 100 and 235 of the Treaty of Rome, along with subsequent amendments to them, have given the EC some room for manoeuvre in developing its competence in relation to occupational health and safety by using general powers. Article 100 (94 in the Consolidated TEU) permits the Council '. . . after consulting the European Parliament and the Economic and Social Committee', to 'issue directives for the approximation of such laws, regulations or administrative provisions of the Member States as directly affect the functioning of the common market' (European Communities, 1997: 75). Article 235 (308 in the Consolidated TEU) allows 'the Community [if it] should prove necessary to attain . . . objectives of the Community and Treaty [for which it] has not provided the necessary powers . . . [and to act] . . . on a proposal from the Commission and after consulting the European Parliament' (European Communities, 1997: 163). Given such Treaty provisions it seems reasonable to suggest that where there is a real European political will there is a way to achieve a common purpose and to concert action to make workplaces across Europe safer and healthier.

There are plenty of specific measures to which the Commission can point – and that is precisely what DGV has done, at its *Europa* web site – as evidence that it has and that it continues to play a significant role in health and safety at work. European Directives and Regulations concerning occupational health and safety adopted or amended since 1978 include measures to:

1. protect workers exposed to vinyl chloride monomer;
2. protect workers against risks related to exposure to chemical, physical and biological agents at work;
3. protect workers against risks related to exposure to metallic lead and its ionic compounds;
4. protect workers against risks related to exposure to asbestos at work;
5. protect workers from risks related to exposure to noise;
6. regulate the sale and use of machines and protective equipment so that they conform with safety requirements;
7. define common essential principles which should be accepted throughout the EC and establish a framework capable of being applied to safety and health in the workplace in all member states;
8. set minimum safety standards for the use of mobile equipment and for equipment used to lift loads;
9. protect workers from risks related to exposure to BSE and TSE agents at work;
10. set occupational limit values for known carcinogens in the workplace
11. set limits to the amount of time that workers can be required to work and about the ways in which working time can be organised;
12. protect specific groups of workers including workers with fixed-duration employment contracts, young workers and pregnant workers and nursing mothers;
13. harmonise laws in Member States relating to electrical equipment used in work environments, where there is a significant risk of explosions;
14. set minimum safety and health requirements for work with display screens;
15. set minimum requirements for the provision of safety and/or health signs at work;
16. set requirements for improving safety and health protection for workers engaged in drilling work;

17. set minimum safety standards for those working on board fishing vessels and arrangements for medical treatment on board vessels;
18. provide for improvements in the collection and publication of information on safety, hygiene and health at work;
19. amend, refine and extend a European schedule of occupational diseases;
20. establish a Scientific Expert Group (SEG) to give advice on setting limit values for risky materials and substances in the workplace and incorporate the work of the SEG – through a Scientific Committee on Occupational Exposure Limits (SCOEL) – into Commission proposals on occupational exposure limits (OELs).

It is hard to resist the impression, given by this list, which is based on just some of the material published by the European Commission about its occupational health and safety legislation, that the EC/EU has become a major player in occupational welfare throughout Europe. Indeed Martyn Davidson, in a review of the legal aspects of work related disorders published in the *British Medical Journal (BMJ)* in 1996, observed that: 'Recent health and safety law (in the UK) has been driven by the European Commission' (1136–40).

Although what the Commission labels the process of transposition may be a slow and difficult one, Davidson concludes that: 'Domestic legislation is generally enacted to fulfil the requirements of (EC) directives.' And he goes on to point out that it is open to the Commission to take member states that fail to transpose (to reflect EC Directives in their domestic legislation) to the ECJ to force them to do so.

This is not a method much favoured by the Commission. The Commission has been keen to proceed in ways that rely on the willing consent of member states and on social dialogue across Europe and within individual member states. Processes it seeks to support by obtaining and issuing expert opinions, work safety findings and a range of comparative data. This strategy, which seems to fit well with the model at the heart of EURATOM involves a variety of EU-sponsored bodies: SCOEL (referred to above), the EASHW, the European Foundation for the Improvement of Living and Working Conditions (EFILWC), SLIC (the Senior Labour Inspectors, Committee – which provides a European forum for senior staff involved in national health and safety inspection work), and the Advisory Committee for Safety, Hygiene and Health Protection at Work (ACSHH). These are Commission-sponsored bodies which are clearly designed to build partnerships, create consensus and disseminate key findings about dangers in the working environment and to improve the effectiveness of health and safety legislation. The principal Commission anxiety – which is clearly evident in Commission literature – is that employers, large employers but most especially small employers, will resist health and safety legislation and the harmonisation of existing measures because they believe that EU regulation and law-making will undermine competitiveness and add to costs.

Getting everyone working together

The EASHW has, since its establishment, worked hard to challenge the idea that attempts to harmonise health and safety measures and the adoption of the highest standards of health and safety in the workplace, throughout the EU, will undermine competitiveness and add to costs. This is a point to which we will return. Having operated informally since 1982, as a 'Group of Senior Labour Inspectors', the Commission announced in July 1995 (Commission PR, 1995) that it was establishing a SLIC consisting of representatives of the labour inspection services of the member states. SLIC would help the Commission to achieve 'correct transposition' of health and safety legislation. SLIC, the Commission went on to assert, would enable the Commission to 'promote the greater involvement of the 9,000 labour inspectors in the 15 member states in encouraging the effective enforcement of Community law'. SLIC would give 'opinions on problems relating to enforcement by the Member States . . . [and enable the] . . . Commission . . . to develop the necessary initiatives in [the] field'. Such an arrangement, with SLIC meeting regularly, was consistent – it was suggested – with the principle of subsidiarity. Member states would be free to do what they could do best while the Commission and the European institutions which it served could play their full part – in an informed way – in making workplaces throughout the EU safer (Commission PR, 1995).

Incorporating specialists and professionals, likely to share Commission goals, from across the EU, seems to be a very attractive strategy for a supranational body that has modest resources of its own. ACSHH has played a major part in the European *Action Programmes* which have helped launch and sustain the EU health and safety legislation and the Commission's expanding health and safety competence. It has some 90 members – last nominated in July 1997 to serve until July 2000. The Committee adopted an ambitious and wide ranging programme of work, for which the Commission can claim considerable legitimacy, given the Committee's make up and method of appointment. It consists of two government representatives, two trade union representatives and two representatives of employers from each member state. They are appointed by the Council – the institution that embodies the authority of member state governments. The Advisory Committee is itself an embodiment of notions of social partnership and social dialogue – the base for EC consensual law making in the social field.

In October 1997, at its 55th plenary meeting, the Committee adopted proposals to: advance work on risks related to exposure to carcinogens at work; support the idea of applying legislation on health and safety at work to self-employment; support a draft Directive concerning medical care on board vessels and develop legislation to regulate display screen equipment. The Committee also gave its backing to a third European week on health and safety, which took place in 1998, approved the 21st annual report on its activities (for the year 1996) and gave its blessing to the work programme of the recently established EASHW. It also laid down a work programme that included combating violence at work and the development of better health-management systems. The Committee, which requires an absolute majority to make policy (which it does by issuing opinions), cannot be said to be lacking in ambition. The Committee is chaired by a member of the European Commission and serviced by the Commission.

Another body that appears to reflect the Commission's determination to make investments in intellectual partnerships as well as social partnership and dialogue is the EFILWC. When the Council of Ministers decided to establish EFILWC in 1975 it was intent on creating an intellectual resource capable of helping Europeans plan and introduce improvements in the workplace and beyond (EEC Regulation No. 1365/75, Council, 26 May 1975). The Foundation, located in Dublin, was specifically directed by the Council to focus attention on the best ways of improving conditions for:

- 'Man at work';
- 'The organisation of work and particularly job design';
- 'Addressing problems peculiar to certain categories of workers';
- 'Considering long-term aspects of improvement of the environment'; and,
- 'The distribution of human activities in space and in time'.

The European Foundation is expected to collaborate closely with institutions that are concerned with the working environment in all member states and itself proclaims its determination to be an active member of the recently established European Network on Work Organisation (EWON). EWON has been set up by the European

Commission in response to its Communication on 'Modernising the Organisation of Work – a Positive Approach to Change' (1999). It is notoriously difficult to measure influence, intellectual activity and output but the Foundation's publications unit estimates that it produces over 60 titles a year, in different languages, on paper and electronically. Judged by such criteria it appears to have been serving its purpose.

The European Agency for Health and Safety at Work (EASHW)

The EASHW is based in Bilbao, Spain. It began its work in 1996, having been made possible by two Council Regulations agreed in 1994 and 1995 (2062/94 and 1643/95). The Agency's objective, set out in the founding Council Regulation, is 'to encourage improvements in the working environment'. In order to bring about improvements the Agency is expected to 'provide (European) Community bodies, the Member States and those involved in health and safety work with the technical, scientific and economic information' they need to promote safety and health at work. The Agency is expected to build on Treaty commitments and 'successive action programmes concerning health and safety in the workplace'. The Agency Director is accountable to an Administrative Board made up of representatives of government, employers and workers from the 15 member states of the EU along with representatives of the European Commission.

In *Building the Links,* the Agency's glossy introductory account of its role and activities, it identifies a series of responsibilities for European working environments that echo Articles at the core of EURATOM Treaty (EASHW, 1998a: 1).

As the Agency puts it ... Guided by the needs of its users it will:

- provide access to information about best practice from a wide variety of sources;
- facilitate the exchange of experience of practical solutions to common problems;
- analyse and disseminate information about important safety and health subjects;
- tailor its different information services to the user;
- contribute to future European Community programmes;
- build two-way information links with Community bodies and organisations throughout the world;
- aim to include the principal organisations and national bodies in the area of health and safety in its network;

- encourage health and safety bodies to contribute to and benefit from the 'Information Society'.

In the first reports it has commissioned and published the Agency has sought to meet head on the kinds of questions that are a frequent counterpoint to the establishment of yet another EU body. Is it necessary? Can it do anything worthwhile to improve health and safety in the workplace? Is it appropriate for the EU to seek to develop its legislative and standard setting role any further? Is another European Agency the right way to do it?

The Commission itself, in reviewing its work programme covering the period 1996 to 2000, appeared to be responding to just these kinds of questions. Questions which increased EU action on health and safety at work might naturally attract from sceptics, particularly the Euro-sceptic British, who doubt that the EU can add much to member state initiatives and actions.

At the top of the Commission's list of priorities for health and safety at work – up to 2000 – was 'Making legislation more effective', next came 'Preparing for enlargement' (DGV, 1999c; EASHW web site). The EU is planning for additional member states, who anticipate considerable difficulties in satisfying existing EU Directives and Regulations on occupational health and safety. The Commission clearly believes that, given the determination among existing member states to move to enlargement, it has a very demanding role to play in preparing for and helping to implement a pre-accession strategy for would be member states. As concerns its top priority – effective transposition – the Commission has recently estimated that some 95 per cent of European health and safety legislation has now been transposed and argues that it is necessary and desirable to speed up the process in future (DGVc, 1999). This rate of transposition is itself presented as evidence of effectiveness and a justification for further investment in advancing harmonisation. If member states agree additional measures or amendments of existing ones don't they want to see them quickly and efficiently transposed? Isn't speedy and effective transposition congruent with the creation of a truly common market – limiting social dumping as rigorously as possible?

The other two priorities, in its mid-term work programme review, are: 'Strengthening links with employability' and meeting the challenge of 'Working conditions in a time of change'. The latter is focused on anticipating and identifying new risks in the workplace.

The Commission justifies the first of this pair of priorities with reference to a Eurostat European Household Panel Survey. The survey found that about 17 per cent 'of the (EU's) working age population regarded themselves as being severely or to some extent hampered in their daily activities by a chronic physical or mental health problem, illness or disability' (DGV, 1999c). If substantial numbers of individuals (and an earlier Eurostat estimate from 1991/92 put the figure of those hampered to some extent at 10 per cent) have a reasonable fear of exclusion from the labour market then the Commission argued a considerable EC effort was needed to ensure good access to employment and contain the risks of social exclusion. All who want to work should be able to. Doesn't this require concerted action across the EU – most particularly if social dumping is to be avoided? On the second point the former Commissioner for Employment and Social Affairs, Padraig Flynn, told a Conference, held in Bilbao, shortly after the opening of EASHW that: 'Manufacturing now accounts for only 20 per cent of total employment and even within manufacturing, workers are more likely to be in front of a computer screen rather than a blast furnace' (EASHW, 1997).

The Commissioner was advancing a theme of European policy-makers, which is reflected in much contemporary debate about work and welfare. The changing world of work makes it essential for those concerned with occupational health and safety to inform themselves about what is changing and what needs to be done to adapt legislation and practice to altered working environments and contracts of employment.

It has to be acknowledged, however, that good intentions and detailed legislation do not, by themselves, guarantee effective action. Transposing European Directives does not provide an assurance of 'effective implementation' or 'practical application' in member states (DGV, 1999c). This is where the Commission and its Agency in Bilbao are required to play a critical part. The Agency is expected to develop the means to help evaluate the effectiveness of existing legislation for health and safety in the workplace. It is also expected to develop and disseminate the evidence and arguments that employers, most particularly owners and managers of Small and Medium-sized Enterprises (SMEs), in fiercely competitive markets, will find convincing.

The principal elements in the European Commission's strategy for developing the EU's occupational health and safety role can be organised under five main headings:

- Communicate the scale of the issues involved and, in doing so, emphasise the economic, not just the human impact, of unsafe and harmful working environments.

- Deploy the most effective arguments possible to convince businesses, of all sizes, that it makes good business sense to invest in the safest most risk free working environments possible.
- Collect much better data – on accidents, risks and the effectiveness of safety legislation and enforcement regimes – which will permit detailed comparisons between member states and enterprises.
- Make the maximum possible use of contemporary information technologies to disseminate data on accidents, workplace safety and effective interventions that can be shown to reduce risks and make the workplace safer.
- Recruit and involve, in European health and safety work, as many of the key players in member states as possible.

The strategy is unmistakable, when the proposals, work plans and publications of the Commission and its Safety and Health at Work Agency are examined.

In what it describes as its 'first major information project', *Priorities and Strategies in Occupational Health and Safety,* published in 1998, the European Agency presents a detailed and carefully researched case for concerted action to implement the occupational health and safety priorities of member states. The information project was designed to find out directly from member states what their priorities in occupational health and safety were and to identify the ways in which they believed activity at EU level could be most helpful to them. Among the 32 conclusions listed at the end of its report the Agency affirms support for the role of legislation. It claims that there is a widespread desire to improve methods to assess the effectiveness of legislation and of health and safety training, and an acceptance of the need to target high risk areas at work and to improve risk assessment in the workplace. It lodges these conclusions – alongside the substantial support it detects for improving and strengthening arrangements for exchanging information and for sharing experiences between member states.

The European Agency has had little difficulty in assembling data which shows both the numbers and economic costs of work related disease and accidents to be substantial. In its *Building the Links* it asserts that 'every year 6,000 European workers lose their lives as a result of accidents at work'. Readers of this Agency publication are also informed that 'nearly 10 million (people) suffer work accidents and occupational diseases'. The costs fall on individual workers, their families, the communities of which they are a part, member state governments and employers. The costs to employers have been highlighted by the Agency at a series of European conferences on occupational health and safety that it has sponsored and supported.

Conference and conference session titles include: 'Good Safety and Health Is Good Business for Europe' (EASHW, 1997), 'Safety and Health at Work as a Factor for Increasing the Competitiveness of European Business and Health' and 'Safety Measures and Their Social and Economic Impact' (EASHW, 1998d). The latter, a session at a conference organised jointly by interested parties in Europe and the US. In its second major report (1998c), *Economic Impact of Occupational Safety and Health in the Member States of the European EU* EASHW presented evidence obtained from member states which showed the costs to society of work-related injuries and ill-health estimated as a percentage of Gross National Product(GNP):

> Although varying methods of calculation exist in different Member States, as a general rule, these estimates ranged from 2.6 per cent to 3.8 per cent of GNP. This would indicate a total cost of between EU185 billion and EU270 for the EU as a whole. (These figures are comparable to the estimated GDP for 1999 of Austria and Belgium of EU198 billion and EU214 billion respectively.)
>
> (EASHW, 1998c)

The European Commissioner, Padraig Flynn, seized upon the report as an opportunity to press home the point that 'the case for better health and safety standards in the workplace will be strengthened if policy makers are better informed of what poor standards actually cost and how these costs can be reduced' (Commission PR, 1999b).

In his presentation to the European Agency's conference, 'Good Safety and Health Is Good Business for Europe', Dr Bodo Marschall, an employer representative from the German car manufacturer Volkswagen, claimed that Volkswagen's investment in making the workplace safer had been a very considerable economic benefit to the company. In his presentation, entitled 'The competitive advantages of high levels of health and safety and work' he offered evidence to show that:

> Thanks to technical and conduct-related measures, it was possible to reduce the number of industrial accidents from some 5,500 in 1987 to around 1,100 in 1996. The working days lost have been reduced from around 61,000 to approximately 15,000. Even if one assumes a cost of only DM 500 per working day lost, a very conservative figure, the reduction in costs achieved is immediately apparent. . . . Occupational health and safety helps to maintain and promote the ability and

willingness of our employees to perform their tasks. At the same time, it also makes an important contribution to profitability.

(EASHW, 1997)

The EFILWC (1997b), which has been strongly encouraged by the European Commission to collaborate closely with the EASHW, published the results of a second European survey of working conditions in 1997 (the survey itself took place in January 1996). The survey examined the views of some 15,800 workers from all over Europe – 1,000 workers being interviewed in each member state. The report makes a significant contribution to the development of data resources intended to facilitate comparisons of work related risks and working environments in EU member states. The Foundation's research on working conditions is complemented by its publication, also in 1997, of what it described as 'a tool for policy makers', the *European Working Environment in Figures* (EFILWC, 1997). The report contains recommendations 'for future activities to improve both the working conditions and the monitoring thereof in Europe'. The European Commission's DGV has itself been seeking to develop the means to compare data on accidents at work in different parts of the EU. In February 1997 the first results of a scheme known as European Statistics on Accidents at Work (ESAW) were published reporting on absences from work of more than three days (in 1993) and fatalities at work (DGV, 1999c). The Commission has been making considerable efforts to harmonise data on health and safety at work and to develop European statistical expertise in dealing with occupational health and safety data across the EU. The European Agency will undoubtedly be playing an increasingly important role in this area, so that the quality and exchanges of assessments of effectiveness and economic impact of occupational health and safety measures are improved.

In its 1998 work plan the European Agency made great play of its determination to communicate speedily and effectively throughout the member states. It plans to do this in two main ways. They are closely linked and are designed to integrate the two remaining elements of the strategy identified above. In the European Agency's first edition of its *European Health and Safety Newsletter*, published in February 1998, the Agency explained that:

The Internet was selected as a primary tool to meet the Agency's information distribution objectives. The Internet medium will enable the Agency to deliver up-to-date relevant information to a large audience of users. . . . On [our] homepage, there are 8 main information categories, which display information at the European and national level with the majority of the Member States having their own national pages. . . . The organisations that make up the Agency network consist of the Agency itself and a designated national Focal Point from each of the Member States. All key OSH (Occupational Safety and Health) organisations will also be represented on the system. This network provides one central access point to European occupational safety and health information. . . . A special Internet Group has been set up by the Agency, consisting of national experts from each Member State as well as Agency staff. This Group will manage the network and plan the future development of the network.

For small organisations and units, such as the European Agency, the Commission staff working on health and safety issues within DGV in Brussels, the EFILWC, influence and effectiveness depend on finding, motivating and keeping partners who have access to much greater resources and who share the same interests and goals. The communities of experts and health and safety specialists, including European safety inspectors, are mostly well connected with – to employ the Euro jargon – national Focal Points. The social partners and the networks of expert and specialist officials in member states have the potential to build and sustain a momentum for Commission proposals presented to the Council of Ministers. A momentum which the Commission's principal occupational health and safety staff hope and believe that member state governments will find it hard to resist. That should not obscure the fact that the Commission finds itself giving the impression of walking on a tightrope. It is seeking to balance its commitment to strengthening European health and safety actions while taking account of the politics of shaping proposals which will be acceptable to member state government representatives, who themselves have to satisfy many different and often opposed interests.

The embryonic condition of the pan-European statistical systems for comparing member state accident and health records and evaluating legislation, means that it will be some time before reliable detailed answers are available to reasonable questions about the value and effectiveness of European occupational health and safety legislation. No doubt that is why the European Agency's Thematic Network Group on National Priorities and Programmes observed, in introducing its review of the economic impact of Occupational Safety and Health (OSH) in the member states, that even though 'estimating the costs and benefits of (OSH) measures had become an important issue in most Member States

. . . stress (is placed on) the importance of ethical considerations when it comes to formulating OSH policy' (EASHW, 1998b).

Health and safety at work – a politically charged subject

One thing is clear, as has been well illustrated in the UK by reaction to attempts to apply the Working Time Directive to junior hospital doctors employed by the NHS. Occupational health and safety measures can be, in political as well as economic terms, highly combustible. In an editorial written in April 1996 the *British Medical Journal* observed that: 'The death of a junior hospital doctor in Britain last year, after working excessive hours and sleeping little, brought new relevance to the question, can overwork kill?'. The editorial went on to note that 'empirical research . . . suggests that higher workloads do increase disease and death rates' (Michie and Cockcroft, 1996; see also Ferriman, 1999). In May 1999 the BBC reported that a meeting of European employment ministers was about to hear that the British Government wanted junior hospital doctors to continue 'to work up to 65 hours a week for the next eight years' and remain 'exempt from the European working time directive which orders that employees should not work more than 48 hours a week.' (BBC online, 1999b,d,e,f). The intensity of the subsequent political exchanges, including what the BBC described as the *furious* response of junior hospital doctor's representatives, and the new Labour Government's alleged reluctance to accept an EC proposal to introduce a 54 hour a week limit – in place of the 65-hour one – serves to underline just how fraught the EU role in occupational health and safety can be.

3
Professions and Mobility in Europe

A Europe without borders for workers

Citizens of the EU are entitled to travel to any other EU country – to live, to study *and* to work. With unimportant exceptions, EU citizens are entitled to be treated by employers and public bodies, in other EU member states, in exactly the same way as the nationals of the country where they wish to settle, study or work. Considerable effort has been invested by the European Commission in making it possible for EU citizens to travel, in search of work, throughout the EU. The process of guaranteeing unfettered access, for European citizens, to labour markets throughout Europe has also been supported by the ECJ, in a series of judgements which have entrenched rights of access to employment, irrespective of nationality, throughout the EU (Nielsen and Szyszczak, 1997: 65–135). Difficulties do remain, indeed difficulties with the mutual recognition and transferability of professional qualifications have been identified as the source of the 'most common problems experienced by intending migrant workers within the [European] Single Market' (DfEE and DTi, 1997: 1). But in terms of European law and EU regulations health care professionals now have a realistic expectation that their skills and qualifications will be recognised and accepted anywhere in the EU.

Despite this the impact of the world's largest single market for workers, not just goods and services, on European medical care systems, has been modest. It has been suggested, for example, that:' . . . many designated authorities (concerned with mutual recognition of qualifications across member state boundaries) lack experience of the process, as a result of so few applications being made to them' (Ludvigsen and Roberts, 1996: 123–4). And, to take the British case, the numbers of EC doctors granted full registration has historically run well behind the numbers drawn to the UK from outside the EU (Stacey, 1995: 133). Nevertheless, member states of the EU are all committed to the free movement of workers – including the key professional workers employed by Europe's medical care systems. Yet professionals who move from one member state to another, to practise their profession, are very much the exception rather than the rule. Indeed the small scale of labour flows between EU medical care systems (McKee *et al.*, 1996: 270–4) may appear surprising, in view of the healthy appetite that medical care systems have for trained labour – including labour drawn in from abroad – when professional shortages are encountered. The heavy reliance, which has characterised the British NHS, for example, on medically qualified personnel recruited from 'overseas' – essentially Commonwealth countries – illustrates the point very well (Smith, 1980; 1; Stacey, 1995: 132–3).

Limited mobility in the EU – will it always stay this way?

Medical systems are labour hungry systems. Health professionals, employed in EC countries, taken on their own – and they are far from being the only employees of European medical-care systems – have been estimated to account for 4 per cent of the entire EC working population (Berlin, 1992: 3). Applying Berlin's estimate to Statistical Office of the European Communities (EUROSTAT) figures for the total EU labour force at the end of the 1990s suggests that health professionals, at work in the EU, numbered at least 6 million (EUROSTAT, 1998). And labour is the principal factor of production used by medical-care systems. It accounts for between 50 per cent and 75 per cent of medical system costs and most of the variation in costs between medical systems (Saltman, 1997: 239). What is more, medical-care systems need to constantly replenish their supply of labour – most especially professionally qualified labour. In other words they require a continuous supply of new recruits, many of whom are costly to train. A high proportion of these are to be found among the most able school leavers; young people who do not lack career choices.

Against this background the apparent absence of concern, in the EU, about free-riding may seem surprising. Free-riders, in this sense, can be defined as medical-care systems and member states that set out to employ doctors and nurses, trained elsewhere, in order to keep their own labour costs down. Medical-care systems that look to make use of professionals, trained abroad – to ease the problems of planning and managing their medical service are to be found in the EU (Saltman, 1997: 242–43). However, free riding, in medical-care labour markets, has never been identified as a EU problem, even if some member states, such as the UK, have been criticised for relying unduly upon large numbers of doctors trained outside of Europe. Rather concern in EU countries has tended to focus on finding ways to limit the numbers of university places available to nationals who want to qualify as doctors (Saltman, 1997, 239–41; Mossialos and Le Grand, 1999: 119–21). It is, nevertheless, indisputable that the scale of planning and investment needed to anticipate and meet demands for the most expensive medical system resource of all, skilled health-care workers, is substantial. It is also unarguable that unanticipated professional migration is capable of severely testing, even disrupting a medical-care system's ability to deliver services. Should we – can we – therefore conclude, from the absence of concern or complaints from member states about doctors and nurses, who mount their bikes and take their qualifications elsewhere in the EU, that EU commitments to the free movement of professional labour are of little practical significance? It would be premature to do so.

On considering what may change

It is central to this chapter and the viewpoints presented in it that the potential significance of EU commitments to the free movement of workers – most especially health professionals – should not be underestimated. The consequences of EU laws and regulations, governing the mobility of workers, should not be judged solely on the basis of their impact to date. In making an assessment of the long-term consequences of EU labour mobility regulations, it is advisable to consider the possible future impact of treaty provisions and Commission Directives. EC Directives have met an increasing number – though by no means all – of the important requirements for the establishment of a pan-European labour market for the services of doctors and nurses and their co-workers. The commitments to free movement of workers, embodied in the Treaty of Rome and the SEA, represent a means for releasing powerful – but, for the present, largely latent – forces capable of shaping and influencing the organisation and costs of European medical-care systems. Employers and managers, in member state medical care systems, are now able to look beyond the boundaries of their own national labour markets and within the member states of the EU for the labour they need. It is not difficult to imagine circumstances in which a growing number of them will have an active interest in doing so.

Most legal and technical problems – as this chapter will show – previously encountered in recognising professional qualifications gained in other member states – have been resolved or are now capable of resolution. Health-care professionals themselves may find good reasons to become more mobile in future – in their search for better pay, better working conditions and enhanced professional opportunities. Indeed, the European Commission, in removing or lowering barriers to increased professional mobility, has sought to involve the health professions in EU policy-making. This may itself prove to be of considerable significance in the longer term. Should professional mobility increase it seems reasonable to envisage professional alliances, formed among the doctors and nurses who have moved or who are willing to move, between medical-care systems in different member states, playing an increasingly influential role in setting standards and determining how services are organised. Such alliances of professionals would be concerned not only with payment for their own services but also with the adequacy, range and quality of medical services. Alliances of this kind might find it possible to influence public opinion in member states and even tread a European stage to promote views about the condition and prospects of European medical systems.

Freedom of movement for European citizens – including the freedom to live and work in any part of the EU, not just to travel freely within the EU – is one of four fundamental freedoms guaranteed by the Treaty of Rome and confirmed by the SEA. The freedom to seek and take up employment anywhere in the EU remains untested by most European citizens because obtaining a job, which provides an adequate livelihood, is generally much easier at home, in an environment that you know. Going abroad is likely – even in the freest of labour markets – to add considerably to the difficulties of finding a job. Those difficulties are likely to be increased substantially – even if the employment being sought does not require special skills or qualifications – if the would-be migrant cannot speak the language or does not understand the culture of the country in which he or she wishes to gain employment.

Mutual recognition of qualifications

Although the framers of the EEC appreciated the difficulties they were nevertheless determined to ensure that it would be possible for citizens, coming from any member state, to enjoy the same rights and opportunities, in another member state, as the citizens of that state. A common market needed good foundations. If they were secure, the founders of the EEC seem to have reasoned, others – EC citizens themselves – could be relied upon to make the most of the opportunities provided. The Treaty of Rome (Articles 48–66) made it clear that the freedom, to take up employment in another member state, should not be undermined or jeopardised by special requirements that did not apply to ordinary nationals of that member state. But it was not a simple matter for the Commission to remove barriers faced by workers moving from one member state to another. Ensuring the mobility of workers with professional qualifications posed particular problems. When it was set up in 1958 the EEC lacked any means of establishing the equivalence of professional qualifications gained in different member states or ensuring that jobs requiring professional qualifications were open to qualified citizens, regardless of the Community country from which they originated. It took almost 18 years for member states to assent to the Council Directives, issued in June 1975, which established a framework for the mutual recognition of medical qualifications (75/362/EEC and 75/363/EEC). Agreement only became possible when the European Commissioner, Ralf Dahrendorf, 'cut the Gordian knot by declaring that, whatever their educational background, doctors throughout the Community had similar skills and attributes and . . . qualifications awarded by one member state should be regarded as satisfactory by all the others' (Brearley, 1992b: 30). Frustration with its original attempts, to develop the means to ensure mutual recognition of skills and qualifications, not only influenced Dahrendorf to object to a methodology, for mutual recognition, which necessitated establishing precise and detailed equivalencies for national qualifications. Dahrendorf also emboldened the Commission to develop other approaches to mutual recognition of skills and qualifications. A process strongly encouraged by the passage of the SEA in 1986. The SEM, which is defined in the SEA (which itself came into force throughout the EEC in July 1987), provided much of the impetus to refine and develop the arrangements for mutual recognition of professional qualifications. The Single Market is an area currently comprising the 15 member states of the EU (to which can be added, for most purposes, the European Economic Area states of Norway, Iceland and Liechtenstein). The Single Market does not permit internal frontiers and entrenches the free movement of persons as well as goods, services and capital. An EC deadline for its completion, by 31 December 1992, predated its general adoption, which had been agreed in Luxembourg in December 1985 (Nugent, 1994: 453).

The considerable difficulties, encountered in developing a consensus about professional standards and training needed for the mutual recognition of medical and architectural qualifications made it a priority, for the Commission, to find ways of simplifying the process for establishing mutuality in respecting the professional and vocational qualifications that had been gained in different member states. The freedom of movement, required by the SEM, has in fact been advanced by two additions to the Commission's original approach. They are designed to enable virtually any European citizens, in a regulated occupation or profession, to transfer their qualifications and skills from one member state to another.

The EU now has three systems for the mutual recognition of qualifications and skills; they are based on:

- First General System Directives
- Second General System Directives
- Transitional Measures Directives

In its booklet, *Europe – Open for Professions*, the UK's Department of Trade and Industry, offers an account in plain English of both the philosophy and practical application of each of the systems for Britains who are thinking of exercising their 'freedom to work within the Single Market' (DfEE & DTi, 1997: 1–17).

The First General System Directives, known as Sectoral Directives, apply to doctors, dentists, pharmacists, midwives, general nurses, veterinary surgeons and architects. The Seven Sectoral Directives were issued to cover these professions, following very lengthy and detailed negotiations about the content, comparability and harmonisation of professional training in all the member states. The Sectoral Directives represent an approach that was subsequently abandoned (for all but lawyers) because, in the words of the DTi's guidance to British professionals, it was 'unacceptably complex and slow'. The Second General System Directives, known as the First and Second Diploma Directives (89/48/EEC and 92/51/EEC), were intended to cover all the regulated occupations, professions and titles not covered by Sectoral Directives or by Transitional Measures Directives. They are now known as the General System, for mutual recognition of qualifications. They rest on the premise that any individual, qualified in one member state for a particular profession or occupation, should be accepted as qualified to do the same work in another member state. Aspirations to harmonise professional training across the EU have been abandoned – although the Seven Sectoral Directives remain in place. Member states, which 'require crafts or trades-people . . . to hold a particular vocational qualification [such as the Meisterprüfung required in Germany] . . .' are obliged, by the Transitional Measures Directives, '. . . to accept proof of a prescribed period of experience by the migrant [worker] in his/her home member state as a substitute for the relevant national qualification'.

The arrangements for ensuring that Transitional Measures Directives and the General System for mutual recognition of qualifications work smoothly rely on so-called competent authorities, in each member state. The designated or competent authority is the body concerned with the regulation of the professional group in the country where an applicant wants to work. It must reach a decision within four months – in the case of the General System – of receiving an application for recognition of a qualification from a European citizen from another member state. It can ask an applicant to either obtain additional professional experience or take a training course or take an aptitude test as a condition of recognition. It cannot require more than one additional condition to be met and it is normally up to the applicant to decide how to adapt to different circumstances and requirements that affect practitioners in another member state. Where it rejects an application it must give a written explanation of its decision and the decision can be appealed to a court or tribunal (see Europa, the Eu's principal web server – 'Citizens first').

Two cases, considered by the ECJ (Heylens ECJ 222/86 and Vlassopolou ECJ 340/89), have contributed to European case law and made it difficult for national authorities to reject the qualifications and ignore the professional experience of nationals from other member states, without good reasons.

In January 1996 the European Commission established what it described as a High Level Panel, chaired by the EU Commissioner Simone Veil, to 'examine the practical difficulties encountered by people when trying to exercise their rights to enter, reside and work in another Member State'. The Panel reported in March 1997. It concluded that, with a few exceptions, 'the legislative framework to ensure free movement of people (was) in place, and the majority of individual problems (could) be solved without changes in the legislation' (Veil, 1997: 3). Indeed, EU Directives now cover: access to employment, recognition of diplomas, protection of personal data, the right of residence in member states, trade union rights, social security entitlements in other member states, taxation and the right to be accompanied/joined by family members in another member state. Although the Veil Report contained 80 recommendations they were almost all designed to raise awareness, among EU citizens, of EU freedom of movement, and to make it easier for citizens to 'make use of their rights'. It is hard to disagree with the Commission's own assessment that statutory rights have been successfully established. It clearly sees its primary role in future as communicating those statutory rights to European citizens in such a way that the EU will become 'a genuine "mobility area" in which freedom of movement is . . . a day-to-day reality for the people of Europe' (EU's web-based guide to its policies: SCADPLUS). It plans to do this by developing the European Employment Services (EURES) Network and by using every means at its disposal to enable young Europeans to get to know and understand each other better and to communicate more effectively in each others languages.

EURES was launched in 1994 and has some 500 Euroadvisers, whose job it is to provide information about: (a) cross-border job offers and recruitment opportunities; and, (b) living and working conditions in other member states, in order to facilitate worker mobility and integration. The Veil Panel singled out the EU's *Citizens First* Campaign as an example of how to promote and explain opportunities for mobility. It reported that almost half a million requests for *Citizen First* fact sheets, about working in other member states, had been received. It was described as a 'well-targeted' and 'practical campaign'. The Commission is now heavily engaged in promoting Simpler Legislation for the Internal Market (SLIM) and *Dialogue*, which is intended to build on *Citizens First*, by establishing contact points throughout the EU for citizens to 'resolve problems arising from (the) application of EU rules on . . . free movement' (DGXV, web site). The Commission is clearly determined to make EURES part of the employment services of every member state and to invest in the greatest possible use of new technologies to 'reach more citizens with job offers across borders' (DGXV, web site).

In February 1999, when Directorate General XV of the European Commission reported on progress with EURES, it was able to point to a EU-wide information and advice system, with a substantial Internet presence since June 1998, which was handling over 500,000 enquiries annually about EU job opportunities. But the High Level Panel Report continues to serve as a reminder of the difficulties confronted, not just the opportunities, in increasing EU worker mobility. The Report noted that only 5.5 million, out of 370 million EU nationals, were resident in member states other than their national home.

Mobility and the obstacles in the road

The reasons for the slow and, to Monnet's successors, what must be disappointing development of a truly pan-European labour market (including a pan-European labour market attractive to health professionals) are not difficult to fathom. The factors that seem likely to nurture and encourage its strong development in the 21st century are also reasonably apparent.

Ludvigsen and Roberts, a nurse and a teacher – both with strong professional interests in European institutions and health policies – have described the mostsignificant barrier to mobility among health workers in Europe, apart from a limited knowledge of other European languages, as 'insularity'. They define this as a fear of the unknown and the unfamiliar and a reluctance to accept other people's cultures; something that they suggest is often a reflection of an unmerited satisfaction with one's own culture. Insularity is not just a British problem – though they consider the British are particularly vulnerable to accusations of insularity (and poor language skills). Insularity is something that can make it difficult to settle *and* to gain acceptance, in another country, even when the language spoken is your own or one that you speak fluently. The examples they give, a Belgian nurse finding great difficulty in getting employment in France, a German hospital which recruited 30 nurses from abroad only to find that 28 had left by the end of the year, illustrate why legally enforceable rights, to live and work abroad, cannot, by themselves, be expected to deliver high levels of worker mobility (Ludvigsen and Roberts, 1996: 143–4).

Health professionals do need to be able to understand and communicate with their patients and co-workers. Ludvigsen and Roberts have a point when they argue that: 'Holiday-level fluency in a language is obviously insufficient for professions where . . . interaction with patients (is) often . . . highly personal and confidential'. Although it should also be pointed out that a linguist's skills are ultimately less important than professional motivation and the ability to learn from experience. Social and economic barriers to labour mobility exist within as well as between countries. We should not lose sight of the extent to which any move in search of work can disrupt family life and threaten friendships and social networks. Limited movement between the labour markets of different member states reflects the limited movement that there has been historically between different geographical regions within member states. Often it is only the collapse of a regional labour market that has resulted in substantial worker migration. By and large Europe's health-care workers are not threatened with mass unemployment or dramatic reductions in opportunities to advance their careers – within the national labour markets with which they are familiar. It is surely unreasonable to expect a sudden increase in professional mobility, which culminates in large numbers of health professionals moving from one member state medical-care system to another. It is much more reasonable to anticipate a gradual increase in professional mobility throughout the EU. That gradual increase, which could lead over several decades, to large numbers of workers moving between member states is likely to depend quite heavily, at least to begin with, on what Ludvigsen and Roberts refer to as 'pioneers' (1996: 143). These are adventurous health-care professionals – with fewer family ties than their fellows who find practical solutions, which can be shared with others, to the professional and human problems encountered in moving from working in one medical care system to working in another.

One substantial obstacle to mobility is undoubtedly lack of knowledge and direct experience of other medical-care systems. Although the lack of European awareness in professional training schemes in Britain is heavily criticised by Ludvigsen and Roberts it can hardly come as a surprise that member state training systems, for health care professionals, are focused on meeting domestic requirements and sustaining local traditions and practices (1996: 127–33). The need to recruit, train and retain professional staff, while keeping within budget, means that nurse educators and employers, responsible for the largest groups of health-care professionals, have few if any instrumental reasons to 'Europeanize the curriculum' as Ludvigsen and Roberts urge them to. Professional and regulatory bodies, in the UK, have done little to address issues that do not have an obvious and immediate relevance to the United Kingdom; indeed they have little reason to lead where others are most unlikely to follow.

One particularly interesting example of British authorities acting in a determined fashion, to reshape professional education and training in the UK to take account of the EU, serves to underline the point that national authorities are keenest to act on EU Directives when they create specific legal difficulties and/or provide opportunities to address problems which are already on high on the domestic agenda. As Meg Stacey has argued: 'The relationship between post-graduate and basic medical education . . . [has] caused the General Medical Council difficulty for many years. It . . . lacked statutory power to control the situation.' (Stacey, 1995: 134–5). The European Commission had expressed its concern that the system of specialist medical registration in the UK 'inhibited the free movement of doctors, discriminating against those qualifying in Europe' (Baggott, 1998: 40). Matters came to a head in 1992 when the Commission threatened legal action against the UK authorities (Stacey, 1995: 134). The Department of Health responded to the requirements of European legislation by instituting a review of postgraduate medical education. Following the publication of the Calman Report (DoH, 1993), the UK Government seized the opportunity, provided by the need to conform to EU mobility Directives, to tackle 'long-standing complaints about the informality and unsystematic nature of medical training in the UK'

(Baggott, 1998: 40). The UK government was able to move on specialist training and promote an NHS in which consultant numbers could be increased. It could do this and make it clear that consultants would be expected to play a greater role in providing medical services themselves; encouraging consultants to devote rather less of their time and energy to directing the medical care provided by junior staff. The Government's response to Calman was also presented as congruent with its commitment to reduce junior doctor hours – a commitment with which it continues a largely unsuccessful struggle.

A clearer road ahead

The absence of widespread enthusiasm in Britain, to seize on all the opportunities for professional development and to make more of the European dimension, reported by Ludvigsen and Roberts, should not be allowed to obscure what seems likely to occur in future (1996: 131–4). There are good reasons to anticipate that things will be different in future. Gradual erosion of insularity – cultural and professional – is most likely to result from developments in EU medical care systems arising from two political imperatives. The imperatives, for EU member-state leaders, are: enlargement of the EU and tighter control of publicly funded medical-care systems, to be effected through organisational changes.

The boundaries of the EU are set to expand eastwards to take in Poland, the Czech Republic, Hungary and Slovenia – and there are many others waiting behind them keen to join. Medical-care systems throughout Europe are being subject to new and tougher budgetary disciplines that are being combined with increased local managerial autonomy. Both these developments seem to be favourable to pioneers (in Ludvigsen and Roberts sense of the word), individuals with skills who are prepared to travel in search of better paid work and greater professional opportunities, and medical service managers – with a strong entrepreneurial streak. The systems which have been developed, over more than three decades, to enable professionals to move, with their qualifications and skills, from one member state to another, should be expected to take on a much greater significance in the Europe of the early 21st century than they have had in the recent past.

The process of extending the horizons and involvement of health professionals in health and health-related issues, at EU level, is likely to be most strongly facilitated by the European Commission itself, in both the short and the longer term. The Commission is keen to get professionals involved in its work and now has substantial experience of getting them involved in research and policy development. Although the Commission has modest human and material resources to deploy, its strategy, as in other areas, seems designed to help stimulate and formulate networks of European professionals, academics and member state policy-makers. Networks made up of people who can help and are motivated to help identify communities of interest and to promote a common EU health agenda.

The Commission will – of course – continue to promote educational and cultural exchanges through programmes such as Socrates, which are intended to provide young European citizens with opportunities to learn about each other and to learn from each other. Opportunities it is hoped will have an influence throughout the lives of increasing numbers of younger EU citizens.

The Commission's activities, in creating and extending opportunities for collaboration among health workers and fostering a climate in which more Europeans are confident about living and working in other member states, will be explored in the rest of this chapter. The reasons for regarding the enlargement of the EU and developments in the management of medical system resources as potentially highly significant for the EU – and likely to lead to greater professional mobility – will also be a focus for the rest of this chapter.

Building collaboration and integration

As part of the work of ensuring compatibility of medical qualifications in the EC a Directive (75/364/EEC), establishing an Advisory Committee on Medical Training within the European Commission, was adopted in 1975. The Committee's terms of reference now appear very ambitious and the abandonment of plans to achieve a detailed harmonisation of medical training throughout the EU have significantly modified its role. A fate that has befallen other professional advisory bodies, such as the Advisory Committee on Training in Nursing, established in 1979. Nevertheless these committees have brought doctors and nurses from across Europe together and facilitated the exchange of views and experiences and encouraged leading health-care professionals to compare arrangements for professional education in different member states. They were among the first developments to have connected the health professions directly with the Commission. They have also served as a focus for professional interests and groups, seeking to influence policy-making at EU level.

Many lobby groups now exist, such as the Permanent Working Group of European Junior Hospital Doctors, which produced a report in 1996 entitled *Medical Manpower in Europe by the Year 2000 – from Surplus to Deficit*, to influence fellow professionals and the Commission (BMJ, 1996b). As Mazey and Richardson put it: 'We see . . . a high degree of interest group integration into the (European) policy process, based upon twin "logics" of organisation and negotiation' (1996: 203–9).

However, policy networks linking the Commission with health professionals and academics throughout the EU have, in recent years, come to rely much more on the greatly expanded role of the Commission in promoting research into health and health-related issues. The same is true of its greatly enhanced role, considered in a later chapter, in promoting specific programmes to tackle threats to public health in the EU. As McKee and Mossialos point out, since the first Medical and Health Research Programme (MHR) was adopted in 1978, there has been a considerable growth in EU research funding and this has resulted in a 'significant increase in projects sponsored and research teams involved' (1997: 49). EU-funded research projects normally require researchers to show that their work will lead to benefits capable of being shared throughout the EU and to entail collaboration among researchers drawn from several member states. Networks built on collaborative research and health-promotion projects are an obvious place to look for future collaborations and collaborators, who understand the benefits of European partnership.

With its eyes firmly on the future the EU has funded an action programme known as Leonardo da Vinci (1995–99). The programme has extended beyond the current boundaries of the EU to take in Hungary, the Czech Republic, Romania, Cyprus, Poland and Slovakia. The most recent full programme, formulated in the mid-1990s was aimed at implementing a vocational training policy in Europe designed to 'encourage quality and innovation in national vocational training systems . . . to increase language skills, to promote equal opportunities . . . and to combat (social) exclusion . . .' (SCADPLUS). The project was initially allocated a budget of over Ecu600 million. Its target groups were: apprentices or young people undergoing vocational training; young workers; graduate students; trainers, tutors or persons responsible for vocational training in enterprises; language teachers or trainers; public decision-makers at local, regional or national level; members of a trade union or an employers' organisation.

A programme that has had even more substantial European funding, Socrates, has been implemented in 25 countries, including Hungary, the Czech Republic, Romania, Poland, Slovakia and Cyprus. The objectives of Socrates have been described by the Commission as:

- promoting the European dimension in education at all levels;
- promoting a quantitative and qualitative improvement in knowledge of EU languages;
- promoting co-operation between institutions in member states' education systems;
- encouraging mobility of students and teachers;
- encouraging the academic recognition of diplomas, periods of study and other qualifications.

Socrates has many different elements, including Lingua. Lingua is a programme intended to improve the teaching and learning of EU languages. Lingua has supported training for language teachers – including intensive training courses; grants for intending language teachers to spend up to a year abroad; the development of new language learning tools and joint education projects for language learning. There may be justified doubts about the quality of some of the work that the Commission has supported but it would be unwise to disregard the potential long-term impact, on European integration and labour mobility, of schemes which have brought nationals from across the Union and from outside it, particularly EU aspirant states from Eastern European, together.

A substantial enlargement of the EU is anticipated before 2005. Of 12 applicants for membership of the EU – mostly Central and Eastern European countries – six are now engaged in detailed negotiations for entry (the Czech Republic, Estonia, Hungary, Poland, Slovenia and Cyprus). Between them these countries have a population of 62.6 million (Partridge, 1998: 60). One of the most striking things about the six states concerned is how far their national incomes, expressed in per capita terms – adjusted to take account of purchasing power parities – fall below the current EU average. The Partridge Report, published in April 1998, using figures from Lionel Barber of *the Financial Times* (5 January 1998), observed that, while the EU 15 member states had an average GDP per capita of Ecu17,300 (per annum), the per capita income in the most economically successful of the leading EU applicants, from Central and Eastern Europe, was Ecu10,100 per annum (59–63). It is surely reasonable to anticipate, as the Partridge Report puts it, that: 'If the employment opportunities in the east remain depressed, there is a possibility that the existing Member States will gain access to skilled professional . . . people seeking work . . .' (Partridge, 1998: 61). More than that there must be a high probability that large numbers of well-educated and well-qualified individuals will be prepared to uproot themselves and their families in search of substantially better pay and employment opportunities in

Western and Northern Europe. In a *BMJ* editorial, published in June 1998, two leading British health economists were reported as challenging '. . . the principle of national self sufficiency (in planning the UK's medical workforce)' and 'pointing to the free movement of labour within the European Union and the fact that several European countries produce substantially more doctors than they employ' (Maynard and Walker, 1997: Goldacre, 1998).

The variability of both nursing and medical workforces within the EU and on its borders is very striking. Elias Mossialos and Julian Le Grand observe, in a study of *Health Care and Cost Containment in the EU*, that: '. . . the numbers of doctors per 1,000 population varies from 4.1 in Spain to 1.5 in the UK' (1999: 121). The proportion of doctors who are classified as specialists also varies substantially from 40.7 per cent of practitioners in Belgium to 68.2 per cent in Sweden (figures for 1994) (Mossialos and Le Grand, 1999: 120). Richard Saltman and Josep Figueras, writing on European health-care reform, for the European Regional Office of the WHO, report that in 1994 the numbers of nurses in the Region varied from: 13.7 in Norway and 8.3 in the Czech Republic, per 1,000 population, to 3.7 in France and 3.0 in Hungary. Italy had 4.7 physicians per 1,000 population and Hungary 3.4, the Netherlands and Ireland had 2.5 and 1.7 respectively (Saltman and Figueras, 1997: 240).

Saltman and Figueras, commenting on the most numerous group of health-care professionals, nurses, suggest that:

> The opening of Europe's borders . . . is creating a new phenomenon. Nurses in Central and Eastern Europe and CIS countries tend to move to richer CEE or western European countries [especially Germany] seeking better wages and conditions [and] some western European hospitals actively recruit foreign nurses, even though locally qualified staff may be unemployed.
>
> (Saltman and Figueras, 1997: 243).

If there is to be a greatly expanded labour market, for health professionals, subject to the free movement principles and Directives of the EU, and a growing number of health professionals, who will find moving between member states highly attractive, it also seems likely to be the case that the trend towards decentralisation and increased managerial autonomy in EU medical-care systems will result in service providers who are strongly motivated to recruit staff from further afield. Decentralisation, a general term widely applied to many medical-care system organisational reforms, is hydra-headed. It is often far from clear whether or not decentralisation embraces privatisation as well as the adoption of new management styles (Saltman and Figueras, 1997, 44–52). If decentralisation is defined as a process in which decision-making moves from a higher political or administrative level to a lower one, from central government to local government, national authorities to local authorities, general managers to unit managers, public servants to contractors, then developments in late 20th century health care systems provide endless examples of decentralisation.

New management styles and health professionals in the EU of the future

Medical-care systems, in the EU, are increasingly characterised by management styles adopted and adapted from the private sector. The 'new public management' promotes a tougher approach to financial management, including individual managerial accountability for achieving measurable objectives and it lauds the beneficial effects of a competitive environment for the delivery of public services. Saltman and Figueras, in their WHO review of European health care reform, drawing on the Osborne and Gaebler's *cri du coeur*, for the reinvention of government (1993), explain that the advantages of decentralisation over centralisation are perceived to be:

- flexibility – in responding to changing circumstances and needs;
- increased capacity to identify and respond quickly to problems and opportunities locally;
- increased willingness to innovate and adopt previously untried methods to solve problems;
- an enhanced ability to motivate workers and increase productivity in the workplace.

Encouraging public service managers to take risks, to innovate and to think the unthinkable, in organising medical services, must surely imply a much greater willingness to accept radical measures to manage and contain the largest part of service expenditure – staff budgets. Increasing conflict between managers, with demanding financial targets and responsibilities, and health professionals, with their personal and professional priorities, seems to be inevitable. If they are to respond to a more competitive labour market and more entrepreneurial types of service management the health professionals may find that it is not in their best interests to put the greater part of their energy into battling things out with local management. That would be a poor strategic choice. The health professions' best bet may be to find ways of harnessing public opinion, throughout the EU, to support the cause of continuously raising health-care standards and improving medical services. Winning support for health-care reforms and measures, which require improvements throughout the EU, is surely the best way to undercut attempts to blunt public expectations about continuing improvements in the standards of medical care and professional service. If public expectations do continue their advance and health workers communicate their enthusiasm to do a good job there will be plenty of well paid work to go around.

4

Pharmaceuticals and the EC/EU

Commerce and medicines

Medicines are very big business. After staff costs medicines account for more of the expenditure of EU medical-care systems than any other budget heading. And pharmaceutical research, medicines manufacture and sales can all be presented as European economic success stories. It is little wonder that the EU and its Commission are deeply involved with pharmaceuticals. The EEC was, after all, established to promote a common market for European manufactures and the manufacture of medicines is an important and successful economic activity in the EU. Of course it is important to appreciate that the word medicines describes not only prescription drugs, which are the principal focus of this chapter, but also the (allegedly) therapeutic substances which are bought and sold, without a prescription, over many a retail counter throughout the EU. They also make a major contribution to the economic well-being of the EU.

The scale and significance of pharmaceutical manufacturing in the EU is relatively easy to convey. The information set out immediately below should leave readers in little doubt about why the operation of pharmaceutical businesses, in the EU, is an important shared concern for a diverse set of public policy-makers. The European Commission has described the pharmaceutical industry in Europe as 'a strong industrial sector which makes a strong contribution to Europe's industrial base' (CEC, 1998c: 2–3).

The EU's medicine makers spent Ecu10 billion in 1997 on research and development (R&D); a sum that was equivalent to the EU's favourable trade balance, in 1997 in pharmaceuticals, with the rest of the world. The retail value of the EU's pharmaceutical market was estimated, by the

Commission in 1998, at more than Ecu90 billion; Ecu57 billion of that sum being accounted for by the pharmaceutical purchases of EU health-care systems. The industry's importance extends to its role as an employer. In 1997 it employed 487,000 people – just over 70,000 of them being engaged in research and the development of new medicines.

Few sectors of industrial and commercial activity have caused the European Commission so many difficulties as the pharmaceutical industry. Even though the establishment of a SEM was to have been accomplished by the end of 1992 the 'special characteristics' of the pharmaceutical industry in Europe continue to make it an especially – perhaps uniquely – demanding sector for the EU's leading open market enforcers. In its 1998 Communication, on the future of the pharmaceutical industry, the European Commission made it clear that it was still striving to establish 'a stable and predictable environment in order to protect the health of patients, to ensure rapid access to the market and to encourage therapeutic innovation' (CEC, 1998c: 1).

It is clear that many of the difficulties that the Commission has found in applying single market principles to the pharmaceutical industry reflect the fact that it is seeking to reconcile open market principles in a highly competitive, rapidly evolving international market, with commitments to public safety and member-state autonomy, in regulating medicines. Certainly the determination to respect national arrangements, for the regulation and purchase of pharmaceuticals, at the same time as applying single market principles, poses very considerable problems.

The contradictory character of the Commission's brief for pharmaceuticals is brought out particularly clearly in a key statement of its multifarious aims, delivered in 1998:

> The purpose of the completion of the Single Market in pharmaceuticals is not just to provide an environment which is favourable for pharmaceutical innovation and industrial development, it is also to improve consumer choices in pharmaceuticals of the required quality, safety and efficacy, at affordable cost.
>
> (CEC, 1998c: 1)

The Commission expressed its concern, on numerous occasions in the 1990s, about what appeared to be the declining international competitiveness of the European pharmaceutical industry. Indeed it has been under great pressure, from Europe's medicine-makers, to formulate policies which recognise and value the industry's economic contribution to European prosperity and employment. Round Table discussions –

involving representatives of the pharmaceutical industry in the EU, major purchasers of prescription medicines and the Commission – held in 1996, 1997, 1998 – illustrate very clearly the kinds of arguments presented to the Commission Directorate, DG III – responsible for Industrial Affairs – by leading representatives of the pharmaceutical industry (IMS, 1996; EFPIA, 1997 and 1998). Directorate General III of the European Commission has in fact sought to justify and explain many of its actions, aimed at realising a SEM in pharmaceuticals, in terms of a restoration of international competitiveness to the European industry. Improved competitiveness will, it is claimed, protect employment and encourage investment in European drug firms. Actions identified as necessary, in a 1994 Communication from the Commission, were presented in 1998 as having gone some way towards arresting the relative decline of the European industry and restoring its international competitiveness (CEC, 1993e; Commission PR, 1994). Those actions were aimed at improving 'Community procedures for the authorisation and supervision of medicinal products', ensuring that it was possible to patent medicinal innovations, most especially in the field of biotechnology, throughout the EU, and 'facilitating access to third country markets' for European medicine manufacturers. The latter goal was – the Commission claimed – being achieved through its work with the International Conference on Harmonisation (ICH) on behalf of the EU. Deals done at the ICH can be seen as a part of the general efforts of the European Commission to enter into Mutual Recognition Agreements (MRAs) with countries outside of the EU. The aim is to assist with the international marketing and recognition of intellectual property rights in new medicines developed inside the EU.

While the Commission claims that it will continue to strive to protect the interests of patients in the EU and to uphold the principle of subsidiarity – so that member state medical-care systems can do their own thing to get value for the money they spend on medicines – it nevertheless stresses that 'the completion of the internal market (in pharmaceuticals) is the single most important step needed to make Europe a more attractive R&D [Research and Development] investment location' (CEC, 1998c: 1). Its ambitions, in relation to the EU's role in promoting a thriving European pharmaceutical industry and getting the best deal for all those who need medicines, imply a remarkable reach for the Commission. Actions to promote the SEM in pharmaceuticals will be complemented by policies designed to shape 'the overall climate in which research and innovation take place' (CEC, 1998c: 1). The Commission refers specifically, in this connection, to improving: access to venture capital; public funding of research; programmes to exploit synergies between academia and industry (as well as between basic and applied research); public understanding and acceptance of new technologies, including biotechnology and gene therapy (CEC, 1998c: 1). However, concerns about the safety, quality and efficacy of medicines (about the need for science to go before commerce), have not been forgotten, they have been underscored by the establishment and growing authority of the EU's EMEA based in London.

The European agency for the evaluation of medicinal products

The EMEA has been in existence since 1995, its establishment having been approved by the Council of Ministers in July 1993 (Official Journal of the European Communities, *OJ*, 1993). EMEA has the power to regulate medicinal products for human and veterinary use throughout the EU. Its job is to police and regulate medicines, notably 'high-technology medicinal products . . . particularly products . . . derived from biotechnology' (*OJ*, 1993: 1). The Council of Ministers intended EMEA to provide for the smooth functioning of the internal market in the pharmaceutical sector, while ensuring that 'decisions on the authorisation of medicinal products (were) based on . . . objective scientific criteria . . . to the exclusion of economic or other considerations . . .'. It was anticipated that uniform and transparent decision-making by EMEA would produce results that were respected by all the member states. EMEA was expected to make decisions capable of accelerating access to the market for new medicines that were safe and effective. The key was to be EMEA's role in undertaking 'a single scientific evaluation of the highest possible standard', which would enable it to give a 'marketing authorisation'. This could be followed by 'a rapid procedure', based on 'close co-operation between the Commission and Member States', to get medicines to the market place. EMEA was intended to show how good science and good commerce could be reconciled (EMEAb).

Scientific rigour and integrity were presented as fundamental to the work of the EMEA. The Council required that 'the exclusive responsibility for preparing opinions, on all matters relating to medicinal products for human use, should be entrusted to the [Agency's] *Committee for Proprietary Medicinal Products* (CPMP) and the *Committee for Veterinary Medicinal Products* (CVMP)', so far as veterinary medicines were concerned (EMEAb). Everything that could be done to make sure that the Agency was scientifically rigorous and independent was going to be done; it was established with a permanent technical and administrative secretariat and the authority to follow up and monitor medicines once authorised (EMEAb). This EMEA role is frequently referred to as *pharmacovigilance*. Indeed EMEA is empowered to undertake 'intensive monitoring of adverse reactions . . . in order to ensure the rapid withdrawal from the market of any medicinal product which presents an unacceptable level of risk under normal conditions of use' (EMEAb). It is also 'responsible for co-ordinating the activities of the Member States in the monitoring of adverse reactions to medicinal products' (*OJ*, 1993). What is more the Agency is required by the Council of Ministers to support and advise the Commission on discharging its responsibilities, along with member states, for 'monitoring good manufacturing practices, good laboratory practices and good clinical practices' (*OJ*, 1993).

This chapter's aims

The two main goals of this chapter should already be apparent from this introduction. They are to describe and analyse the role of the EU and its Commission, in promoting a SEM in pharmaceuticals. First, by providing an account of the winding path that has been followed towards harmonisation in the ethical drugs industry. Secondly, by offering an account of the development of EMEA and its growing impact on the testing and introduction of new medicines in the context of criticisms, from Europe's leading pharmaceutical companies, of the EU failure to make greater progress with the development of a single European market in pharmaceuticals.

The role of the Commission in the face of contradictory expectations

The role of the European Commission, as guarantor of the SEM, and the conflict between its market role, which requires it to advance and promote the cause of economic liberalisation in the sale and purchase of pharmaceuticals, contrasts strikingly with the Commission's other role, as a regulator of pharmaceutical quality, safety and effectiveness. The Commission is called upon to act as defender of the interests of ordinary European citizens – and the medical care systems that serve them – as well as a promoter of European industry. The former role may have the greatest popular appeal but the latter role is strongly influenced by an industry that is known to be well-organised and determined to exert influence in Brussels (Greenwood, 1997: 122–3).

The account offered here is intended to turn a spotlight on the high wire act that EU policy-makers have had to perform in trying to reconcile their numerous responsibilities for safety and access to medicines with obligations to the European pharmaceuticals industry and the ethical drugs manufacturers (EFPIA, 1997: 7). Some of the discussion, towards the end of the chapter, will consider the relevance of a developing academic literature on the regulatory role of supranational bodies and institutions, such as the European Commission and EMEA.

The Commission and EMEA are expected to demonstrate independence from the pharmaceutical industry at the same time as they work with the industry to improve its prospects of developing European products that are world-beaters. Both EMEA and DGIII have pursued strategies which make European legislation, reviews of new products, discussions with industry representatives and adverse findings about therapeutic substances as widely and quickly available as possible. They are making increasing use of the world wide web to do this. Their strategy has made it much easier to write this chapter. It also means that readers, who are particularly interested, in the issues raised here, can readily bring their knowledge bang up to date by visiting key EU web sites – EMEA and others: *http://www.eudra.org/emea.html* and *http://dg3.eudra.org/site_map.htm).*

The requirements for transparency and the desirability of transparency, in all dealings between the Commission, the EMEA, member states and the pharmaceutical industry, set out in a Council Directive (89/105/EEC) of 21 December 1988, have provided a reference point for policy developments in relation to medicines. Even when agreement between the Commission, the industry and member states has been elusive, more information about the nature of differences between them has been placed in the public domain than might be expected.

A single market in pharmaceuticals?

The Commission was set the task, in 1987, by the SEA, of developing and implementing measures to open up the trade in pharmaceuticals. It was expected to act in much the same fashion as in every other European business sector. EEC Directives, already in place, suggested (rather optimistically) that the pharmaceutical sector differed from other sectors in only one really major respect. There was a special need for accurate information. Honesty and transparency were essential if good quality information was to be universally available to the medical-care systems that purchased pharmaceutical products and to patients. Accurate information would mean that medical-care systems could be confident of making medically appropriate purchases. Accurate information about quality, safety and effectiveness, as well as cost, could be presented as satisfying the interests of prescribers and the public that they served. But providing accurate data about such things as side-effects and efficacy, linked to readily comparable information about cost, has proven exceptionally difficult.

The Commission has found enthusiasm for a SEM, in prescription medicines, heavily qualified. Qualified not only by member state governments – anxious not to relinquish the controls that they had over prices – but also by the pharmaceutical industry. Both the purchasers and the makers of medicines reject the idea that a single market, in medicines, can be equated with an unregulated market. Both purchasers and makers of medicines have reasons to be wary about each other's motives and about the consequences of accepting decisions made by international bodies. In fact the Commission has found itself pulled in two very different directions.

A strong case was made by the European pharmaceutical producers for arrangements which enhanced the outstanding contribution which European manufacturers believed they were making to member-state economies. On the other hand complex and widely differing arrangements in member states, intended to secure the interests of publicly funded health-care systems – by constraining drug prices and promoting efficacy and safety – were also presented as too good to lose.

Significant Commission involvement with the pharmaceutical industry can be traced back to an EEC Directive on trade in medicinal drugs issued in 1965. The Commission itself now claims that: 'Since the adoption of the first pharmaceutical directive in 1965, the pharmaceutical legislation of the European Union has constantly pursued two objectives: the protection of public health and the free movement of products' (DGIII-EudraLex: Vol. 1, iii). However Council Directive 65/65/EEC, repeatedly modified since 1965, suggests a conflict of objectives remains. Action to safeguard the public health 'must be attained by means which will not hinder the development of a pharmaceutical industry or trade within the Community' (OJ, 1965). Hindrances to an open trade in medicinal products must be removed and, as the Directive acknowledges, this cannot be achieved without the harmonisation of national regulations and procedures. But the pharmaceutical industry has a special relationship with governments in member states. This has made and continues to make its regulation problematic. It is also widely considered to have characteristics, which cause many to question the appropriateness of applying market principles. It is worth identifying these characteristics and considering how they have complicated the process of developing a single market in pharmaceuticals.

The EU Commissioner, Martin Bangemann, had no doubt that, six years after the deadline for SEM, the single market for pharmaceuticals remained under construction. Something he made plain to industry representatives when they discussed the future of the medicines industry at La Chapelle en Serval (Paris) in December 1998 (EFPIA, 1998: 73–5).

Reasons for being reluctant to accept a SEM for pharmaceuticals

Reluctance to accept market forces and a determination to modify them, in the pharmaceutical markets of each member state, is deep seated and reflects a complex set of factors:

- The widespread belief in government circles, throughout the EU, that unregulated competition can easily compromise the safety and reliability of medicines and that public authorities will be unable to escape blame for any harm that results. It is unlikely that memories of the Thalidomide disaster will fade to the point where European governments will be prepared to see safety issues managed commercially and through the courts, in ways that apply to other industries.
- Beliefs about the vital importance of medicines – which are thought to differentiate them from other products. Medicines are easily presented as life-savers – fundamental to health services. Health services which have been placed outside the realm of undiluted commerce by public policy-makers in EU member states. New medicines – which are the intellectual property of just one commercial organisation – present particular problems for publicly funded medical services. Can public authorities, that have an obligation to meet the costs of medical care – including the costs of life-saving drugs – accept a situation in which they cannot constrain charges for live-saving medicines? Can public authorities declare some medicines off limits because of their cost – especially if they are aware that the producer of a patented product could, in the absence of regulation, use their market position to obtain exceptional profits at the expense of publicly funded services?
- The shared desire of EU governments and the pharmaceutical industry to protect substantial national and commercial interests. Pharmaceutical manufacturers and governments in member states are aware that agreements designed to protect domestic markets may have benefits that they can share. Governments may value and wish to keep and

increase the economic return earned from a successful world-wide trade in drugs. A privileged position for a national medicines purchaser can be represented (or viewed) as part of a scheme to encourage a successful exporter. The success of domestic medicines manufacturers may be reflected in higher domestic investment and employment, which in turn enhances government revenues and contributes to national economic success. Pharmaceutical companies may view a privileged position in their home market as a way of limiting competition, from new or existing producers. They may also point out that they are able to make investment and other financial decisions with greater confidence about the environment in which they will have to operate. The British Pharmaceutical Price Regulation Scheme (PPRS) – an agreement between the UK Government and pharmaceutical companies, which has operated in various forms in the UK since 1954 (Taylor and Maynard, 1990: 8; Malone, 1996: 64) – is one of the best known and clearest examples of the monopsonistic deals which abound in the EU and appear to suit at least some pharmaceutical manufacturers and EU governments.

- The recognition that the purchasers of prescription drugs are not consumers in the ordinary sense of that word. Pharmaceuticals are ordered on behalf of patients by their doctors, doctors who do not benefit directly from what is being prescribed and who look to others – predominantly public authorities and insurers and, to a lesser extent, patients – to pay for what they have prescribed. An unqualified responsibility for the cost of a purchase is generally considered to be fundamental to our ideas about how market relationships work and how they lead purchasers to do their best to obtain value for money. The re-engineering of medical-care systems, in order to encourage greater awareness of costs and benefits, is not expected by policy makers to completely overcome the lack of a direct market relationship in pharmaceuticals between manufacturers and the ultimate consumer. Indeed the very complexity of the third-party arrangements established to control and regulate medicine purchases in the EU extends and deepens the difficulties for public policy-makers wishing to respect single market principles.

- The acceptance that there is a strong case to be made for protecting, even enhancing, intellectual property rights in pharmaceutical innovation and development. Drug companies claim that theirs is a market that requires effective international patent protection if new remedies – breakthrough medicines – are to be brought to market as quickly and efficiently as possible. In an unregulated market place it has been suggested that the considerable costs and uncertainties associated with pharmaceutical innovation would prove a deterrent to investment in R&D. Drugs research would collapse or its results would benefit fewer people. Unless companies that are genuinely innovative and prepared to take risks can be confident of substantial economic rewards for new therapies they will not invest. Genuine innovators need the commercial protection and increased profits that comes with secure patents. Cheap copyists – said to be a particular problem in pharmaceuticals manufacture – must understand that they will enjoy only limited commercial success; the big prizes will be directed to the most successful innovators (Taylor and Maynard, 1990: 12).

- Acceptance of the need for substantial investment – public and private – in the independent production of and regulation of information about medicinal drugs. If buyers cannot be expected to beware – no *caveat emptor* here – then there is reason to make special efforts to establish and maintain independent and unbiased sources of information that can distribute objective data about efficacy and safety. Arguments about market failure – in the face of risk and uncertainty – will be known to those who are familiar with Kenneth Arrow's seminal paper on market failures in medical care (Arrow, 1963). The marketing of medicines can be represented as giving rise to risks and uncertainties, akin to those found more widely in medical care systems; risks and uncertainties which cannot be dealt with adequately by purely market arrangements.

Regulation and conflict – what do we really want?

Jan Leschly, CEO of SmithKline Beecham plc, made the mixed feelings and the frustration of Europe's largest and most research active pharmaceutical manufacturers clear, in Frankfurt in 1996, at the first of the Round Tables convened by the EU Industry Commissioner Martin Bangemann. He told the Round Table, on Completing the Single Pharmaceutical Market, that he wished to congratulate the Commission for its 'tenacity in heading towards the goal of single market' but that 'much remains to be done' (IMS, 1996: 32–5).

Leschly's speech to the Round Table conference praised EU institutions for 'an enormous legislative output' and went on to catalogue what had been achieved: 'We have, most spectacularly, the beginnings of a continent-wide regulatory system for product licensing . . . [which] allows us to start operating across Europe as a whole, rather than having to succumb to the peculiarities – regulatory, cultural, linguistic, or whatever – of individual countries.' EU legislation had, according to Leschly:

- established an agreed framework for the classification of medicines in Europe;
- put in place EU rules about promoting and advertising pharmaceuticals;
- made it clear to ethical drug producers what was required from them in labelling, packaging and supplying information with their products;
- established rules governing the wholesale distribution of medicines; and
- restored some of the intellectual property rights lost because of the increasing amount of time taken to win approval to bring medicines to market.

But, Leschly went on, 'there is a downside'. His company had just revised its strategic plan. The revised corporate plan started by noting that SmithKline considered 'Europe [to be] a hostile and turbulent environment for pharmaceuticals'. Leschly's analysis of the problems faced by companies like his own was uncompromising. The goal of an open European pharmaceutical market, a true SEM, could not be reconciled with the fragmentation of pharmaceutical markets in the EU. Leschly, having praised the Commission for its determination and its part in establishing a legislative and regulatory framework to support a SEM, described this as 'less than half the picture'. The greater part of the picture was a diversity of market places and market conditions that led to problems 'which no other single industry in Europe faces'. Instead of an open market with genuine competition between producers there was a 'a patch-work of different, conflicting, and always national, pricing policies'. Yet the special national arrangements he identified throughout the EU (see Table 4.1) can be squared with the letter of EU law. Even if it is extraordinarily difficult to see how they can be reconciled with the spirit of either the Treaty of Rome or the SEA.

The nature of the Commission's difficulties, in completing the single market in pharmaceuticals, were best explained, at the same Round Table conference, by Alfonso Mattera Ricigliano, Director of DG XV/B of the European Commission. As head of the Division responsible for public procurement in the Directorate and responsible for advancing the cause of a single European internal market Mattera described the 'issue of pharmaceutical prices (as) the pharmaceutical industry's obsession, and, in certain cases, even its nightmare' (IMS, 1996: 36).

Table 4.1 Systems for the regulation of pharmaceutical prices operating in member states in 1996

	CoP	CuP	Del	FPr	GPb	IPC	NeL	PaC	PEC	Pep	Pfc	PPc	PrG	ReP
UK		CuP	Del	FPr	GPb		NeL				Pfc		PrG	
Sweden	CoP									Pep				ReP
Spain	CoP	CuP				IPC	NeL		PEC			PPc		
Portugal	CoP					IPC		PaC						
Netherlands	CoP	CuP	Del										PrG	ReP
Luxembourg	CoP					IPC	NeL							
Italy	CoP				GPb			PaC	PEC	Pep				ReP
Ireland	CoP		Del	FPr		IPC	NeL						PrG	
Greece	CoP					IPC						PPc		
Finland	CoP													
Germany		CuP	Del		GPb		NeL						PrG	ReP
France	CoP									Pep				
Denmark			Del										PrG	ReP
Belgium	CoP									Pep				
Austria	CoP											PPc		

Source: Round Table SEM in pharmaceuticals 1996 (IMS, 1996) – and based on material collected and collated at the London School of Economics.

Key: UK = United Kingdom; ESP = Spain; POR = Portugal; NL = Netherlands; LUX = Luxembourg; ITL = Italy; IRL = Ireland; GR = Greece; FIN = Finland; D = Germany; F = France; DK = Denmark; BEL = Belgium; AUT = Austria.

CoP = Control on Price; CuP = Price Cut; Del = Delisting; FPr = Freeze on Prices; GPb = GP budgets; IPC = International Price Comparisons; NeL = Negative List; PaC = Priced according to Average Price; PEC = Pharmaceutial Expenditure Ceiling; Pep = Pharmaco-economics-based pricing; Pfc = Profit Control; PPc = Priced at production cost; PrG = Promotion of Generic drugs; ReP = Reference Pricing.

There is no EC legislation, he told those present, which denies member states the power to fix prices, 'provided that prices are fixed in a way that does not discriminate – *de jure* or *de facto* – between national and imported . . . products'. Member states can fix the prices of goods if they can claim they have a legitimate purpose in doing so. Included among those purposes Mattera listed: 'protecting the health and life of humans (especially the worst-off social groups), sound social security management, rationalising public finances'. The limitations on such price fixing were that it could not be done, by one member state, in such a way as to handicap imports from another member state. Neither was it acceptable to set prices at an 'unreasonable level'. In the case of medicines, he explained, this meant that such things as research spending, raw material costs, advertising and trading margins had to be taken into account. Member states were, nevertheless, entitled to insist that medicine-makers accepted financial sacrifice, providing they were not being required to trade at a loss. Indeed pharmaceutical companies were, according to Mattera, entitled to expect sales to be remunerative – but the level of remuneration that can reasonably be expected remains ill-defined.

Constraints on pharmaceutical prices are quite lawful then; they can be made consistent with the requirements of the European single market. Purchasers of prescription medicines must – when they constrain the price of pharmaceuticals – do so fairly; they must keep within European law.

The devils that are found in the detail of European pharmaceutical price regulation – and in the uneven and uncertain progress to a SEM in pharmaceuticals – reflect the difficulties that are, it seems, inevitable when operating price controls. Price controls have to be fair and to be seen to be fair but there is no clear or mandatory formula for establishing what is fair. Mattera told his listeners that any method for calculating the prices of pharmaceuticals, imposed by public authorities and social insurance schemes, must be based on criteria that are:

- objective;
- economic;
- transparent;
- verifiable;
- non-discriminatory (this could, he suggested, be true of a method that took account only of parameters specific to the national market); and,
- non-restrictive (this could mean a method that fixed pharmaceutical prices by reference to the lowest price charged in the Community).

(IMS, 1996: 36)

But ensuring respect for the criteria is, as Mattera also explained, a shared responsibility. The pharmaceutical industry must work closely with the Commission. The industry must play a leading role in seeing that all is fair in the medicine markets of Europe. If producers suspect arrangements between major purchasers and a particular medicine seller are inconsistent with the criteria 'it is up to pharmaceutical companies to establish the . . . facts complained of'. Mattera warned the industry against 'passivity or resignation' in the face of 'rule-breaking or abuse'. He had another piece of advice for the leaders of the pharmaceutical industry as well: '. . . you must avoid a "selective policy" . . . (when making complaints). . . . Such a policy creates distortions which will eventually backfire on the European industry as a whole' (IMS, 1996: 37–8).

The complexities of markets for pharmaceuticals, in which member state governments and social insurance systems seek to regulate prices in the public interest, do not end there. They are compounded by the existence of what is known as *parallel medicine imports*. Legal actions, decided in the ECJ, have confirmed the lawfulness of parallel imports. It is legal to purchase prescription medicines in one European country, where prices are low, and sell them in another country where prices are higher. In other words it is possible for middle men, of various descriptions, to make substantial sums by taking advantage of price regulation in the member states that hold pharmaceutical prices down most strongly. Parallel traders are able to undercut producer prices in what are – typically – wealthier medicine markets. The pharmaceutical industry finds itself caught between an interpretation of the SEM, in pharmaceuticals, that permits national price regulation and a legal framework that supports free trade throughout the EU.

An expert observer, Mike Burstall, has asserted that: 'the research-based sector (of the pharmaceutical industry) is particularly sensitive to (the) threat' from parallel traders (1990: 69). Raymond Gilmartin, Chairman of Merck & Co, with a substantial presence in European pharmaceutical production and sales, complained bitterly to CEO's of European drug companies and Commission representatives that, despite vigorous attempts to defend his company's intellectual property rights and set common prices for Crixivan, Merck's AIDs drug, the parallel trade was threatening and undermining his company's ability to establish a common price and assure the profitability of its innovatory research. Gilmartin went on to describe as 'a significant setback . . . a ruling by the ECJ' which had sustained the rights of parallel importers to buy and sell medicines anywhere in the Union (IMS, 1996: 40–1) – something to which we return at the very end of this chapter. Against this background readers may readily appreciate why some pharmaceutical companies believe there are numerous opportunities for misunderstanding and conflict between the industry, member states and the Commission and why they are unlikely to find a smooth path to a SEM (IMS, 1996: 47–8, 61). It also becomes possible to understand why Leschly, in summing up his view on the state of the European pharmaceutical market, claimed that: 'The pharmaceutical industry is simply not at liberty to set its own prices, to set a single price, or, therefore, to operate effectively as if this was a so-called single European market' (IMS, 1996: 33).

Variations in price and use of pharmaceuticals are more complex still

It would be wrong to conclude that variations in the use and price of pharmaceuticals, in different parts of the EU, are simply a reflection of the combined and complex interaction of SEM regulations and diverse medicine purchasing policies. It is much more complicated than that. Variations also reflect – among other things – widely divergent attitudes to medicines and to prescribing them. Saltman and Figueras report German spending on medicines at double the level in the UK. They report differences between spending on medicines in the UK and France which are equally great (1997: 176). The proportion of health expenditure going on drugs in 1993, in EU member states, ranged from over 18 per cent in Spain and Germany – and more than 16 per cent in Belgium and Greece, to less than 12 per cent in Denmark (Organisation for Economic Cooperation and Development, OECD, 1996). In seeking to emphasise how substantial the impact of cultural differences, among physicians and patients, are – on prescribing and consumption patterns in Europe – Burstall was moved to observe that the 'French urge to consume drugs is almost insatiable' (1990: 66). As Burstall went on to explain this should make us cautious about jumping to conclusions about the significance of even markedly different prices for the same drugs in different parts of Europe. As pharmaceuticals are relatively cheap to manufacture – even though they may be very costly to develop – there can be a substantial difference in drug-company earnings from one market to another, depending on the volume of medicines sold. Price is not the only important consideration. High prices may well go with low consumption and vice versa. And one should enter yet another note of caution: the enormous variations in the numbers of pharmaceutical products which can be prescribed, the substantial differences in how they are packaged and dispensed in different parts of the EU, also make comparisons hazardous (Saltman *et al.*, 1998: 261–86; EFPIA,1997: 19). These are differences that are intensified by currency fluctuations.

The industry case – take note of international competition

Notwithstanding the problems of making informed price comparisons the most research active and minded pharmaceutical companies have argued, with some success, that the EU needs to take strong action to protect companies which invest in the development of new drugs. It is suggested that if it does not it will find that it cedes both sales and industry leadership to American drug manufacturers who will increase the concentration of research and development work in North America. It was Pierre Douaze, Head of the Healthcare Division of Pharma Sector Novartis, who did much to sound the alarm about the future of biotechnology research in the European pharmaceutical industry at the Round Table meeting held in Frankfurt in 1996. Douaze identified a huge and growing gap, in the mid-1990s, between US and European biotech companies. Despite its vast market for medicines, he told the Round Table attendees, 584 biotech companies in Europe employed just 17,200 people, compared with the 1,308 US companies which employed 108,000 staff. Douaze claimed that of the top 100 biotech companies 96 were located in the US – just 4 in Europe. R&D spending in the US was the equivalent of Ecu5.9 billion compared with Ecu0.6 billion in Europe. Acknowledging the differences between Europe and the US, in attitudes towards new technologies and the role of entrepreneurship, Douaze argued that public policy in the Union had to address the gap, if the European pharmaceutical industry was not be marginalised internationally. His chief recommendation was an enhanced dialogue between member state governments, the European Commission and the research leaders among Europe's pharmaceutical companies. He anticipated that an enhanced, and better informed, dialogue would lead to an altered balance between the competing objectives in member state health care systems. He was confident that the case for quicker acceptance of new medicines and higher prices for genuine innovations would gain much greater acceptance (IMS, 1996: 13–15; EFPIA, 1997: 10–11). It appears difficult to do anything other than reiterate the conclusion arrived at by Taylor and Maynard in 1990, in their briefing paper on medicines in Europe. There are recipes for success – if we want to get the best out of pharmaceutical firms, capable of producing worthwhile medical innovations (both economically and therapeutically). We should note that '. . . pharmaceutical companies based in intelligently regulated environments (rather than merely protective ones) have been most likely to succeed in global trade' (1990: 23).

However much they protest about the limitations of a mountain of European legislation applied to the pharmaceutical industry, it seems that neither the industry nor Europe's medical-care systems and drug purchasers actually want a truly free and open pharmaceuticals market. What is being sought is a market system where European sub-markets – national markets – are better integrated and offer high returns to pharmaceutical companies that can innovate consistently and successfully. The role of the EMEA, in establishing rules for the sale of new and highly innovative prescription medicines, is now widely perceived to be critical for the future of the most scientifically and technically dynamic of Europe's pharmaceutical firms.

An extended role for EMEA?

Intelligent management of the relationship between major ethical drug purchasers in Europe and pharmaceutical companies is increasingly focused on the quality and transparency of information about medicines. If there is no obvious, simple and local resolution of the problems that arise from trying to reconcile the independence of national drug purchasing agencies with European regulation, and the principle of subsidiarity with the free trade requirements of European legislation, then we need to look to improved European collaboration. Surely the best accommodation of the rival interests of drug purchasers – who want cheap, safe and effective drugs – and producers – who want a reasonable gamble on big commercial prizes from bringing new medicines to market – is to be found in equipping all the parties with high quality information. What might be called institutionalising the spirit of the Round Tables on the single market for pharmaceuticals. This appears to be the conclusion of Claude Le Pen, who was the rapporteur for a Commission Working Group on the single market in pharmaceuticals (EFPIA, 1997: 20–1). Professor Le Pen recommended that the EU establish an 'observatory for pharmaceuticals . . . which should be assigned several tasks'. Those tasks would include the study of price movements, the development of pharmaco-economics and 'expanding knowledge about pharmaceuticals', by providing much improved information about medicines to 'politicians, journalists, and the public at large'. This was to be a key ingredient of policies which would raise the level of understanding 'about what society has at stake in pharmaceutical development' (EFPIA, 1997: 21).

A bid to become the home for such an observatory was speedily lodged by EMEA's Executive Director, Fernand Sauer. Sauer explained that, despite facing 'a very difficult situation' – because of member state reluctance to abandon their legitimate sovereignty in the health field – EMEA had been able, by playing its part in creating 'a network of partners', to achieve considerable progress in the pharmaceutical sector. He explained that, in addition to the national drug licensing authorities, EMEA worked with some 2,200 European experts who made up the network on which EMEA's licensing and pharmacovigilance activities relied (EMEA, 1998b: 9,14). Sauer presented what he described as an 'optimistic view' about collaboration between member states.

It was possible to reconcile a multiplicity of objectives for pharmaceuticals. Sauer claimed such optimism was justified by EMEA's experience and by what the Agency had achieved in less than three years. EMEA had been able to dramatically improve – speed up – access to the market for new drugs. It had been taking 'an average of four to six years' to get new pharmaceutical products fully authorised and into the European market place; EMEA had totally changed the situation. 'Now it takes less than one year to get better products on the EU market' (EFPIA, 1967: 31). EMEA stood 'ready to offer' its skills and success in 'providing high quality information on medicines' to patients, social security authorities, involved in funding the purchase of medicines, the pharmaceutical industry and member state governments. Sauer referred specifically to the proposal made by EMEA's Management Board Chairman, Strachan Heppell, that EMEA become 'active in mobilising networks for better information and more rational use of medicines' (EFPIA, 1997: 31).

EMEA's current responsibilities

The EMEA, established in 1995, describes its main tasks as:

- providing member states and EC institutions with the best possible scientific advice on the quality, safety and efficacy of medicinal products for human (and veterinary) use;
- mobilising multinational scientific expertise in order to achieve a single evaluation system for authorising medicines for sale throughout the EU;
- arranging speedy, transparent and efficient procedures for authorisation, surveillance and, where necessary, withdrawal from sale of medicinal products;
- advising pharmaceutical companies on drugs research;
- co-ordination of pharmacovigilance and inspection activities;
- creating and maintaining the databases and telecommunication facilities to promote more rational use of drugs and ready access for all interested parties to information (EMEAb).

Ethical drugs can in fact be licensed in three ways in the EU. EMEA is responsible for the centralised procedure, under which applications can be made to it directly. EMEA decisions – technically recommendations to the European Commission, for its formal approval – are binding on all member states (SCADPLUS). Biotechnology products have to be submitted to EMEA for evaluation and for a decision on market authorisation. Other new – non biotechnology products – can either be authorised and licensed for sale by EMEA or by national licensing authorities, such as the Medicines Control Agency, which is the UK national body.

It is noteworthy that EMEA has attracted substantial numbers of 'optional applications'. In 1998 it reported that optional new references made up two-thirds of applications for product approval (EMEA, 1998b: 22). In the event of a dispute about a national licensing authority's determination EMEA becomes involved, with the aim of resolving disagreements. EMEA's decision about a dispute is binding. Ultimately it has the authority to approve a medicine, that is the subject of a dispute, for release across the EU. It is also possible for pharmaceuticals to be approved by a national licensing authority for release in the member state concerned alone. EMEA's role and the regulatory apparatus established in 1995 will be comprehensively reviewed sometime in 2001 (EMEA, 1998b: 13).

It is the final task, in EMEA's own listing of its responsibilities (see above), which it is keen to develop further. It is a role – should it succeed – that will put EMEA at the very heart of the conflicts and controversy that surrounds the sale of medicinal products to Europe's medical-care systems.

As numerous contributors to the European Round Tables have acknowledged, EU policy on the free trade in pharmaceuticals runs head on into the determination of member states to retain the instruments of domestic policy, to which the principle of subsidiarity entitles them. Industrial policies formulated with the goal of promoting a strong, profitable, innovative and internationally competitive Europea pharmaceutical industry appear to be at odds with health and social policies, intended to make the very best health care available to all of Europe's citizens. This includes the EU's poorest citizens in its poorest member states.

The development of a highly sophisticated pharmaco-economics, able to distinguish between genuine, therapeutically valuable innovations and other medicines, which may be presented as new and useful preparations but which are neither new nor cost-effective, can convincingly be presented as the best way to overcome – or at least elide – conflicts between industrial policy and health policy. If a respected European Agency can not only develop systems to promote high quality pharmaco-economics but can also manage the rapid dissemination of such information, to member states and prescribers – as well as the third party payers for medicines (public authorities and social security authorities and even patients themselves), it could indeed play a leading role in creating the 'headroom' needed by the most innovative parts of the pharmaceutical industry to obtain high returns for the best new medicines. High levels of profitability, for breakthrough medicines, could more easily be accepted, while other pharmaceutical costs are screwed down. This would enable the best pharmaceutical innovators – so the theory goes – to meet the enormous investment bill for developing new medicines by attracting the risk capital required to be at the cutting edge of pharmaceutical product development.

EMEA is currently working on Medicines Information Network for Europe (MINE) 'to provide better and more accessible information about the efficacy of medicines' (EMEA, 1998b: 10). Strachan Heppell has explained EMEA's aims for MINE as follows:

> to collect and validate information about the efficacy of medicines and make it easily accessible to health care professionals and the public. . . . The results of (a) pilot project . . . will be carefully evaluated . . . MINE . . . will be a co-operative venture, where the Agency's role will be to harness the knowledge and judgement of professional networks across Europe, including universities and public agencies. The EMEA will work closely with national authorities . . . I also hope that the project will involve other key interests, including health care professionals and management, patient and consumer bodies and the industry bodies concerned.'
>
> (EMEA, 1998b: 10).

EMEA's successes in developing an effective regulatory role are generally acknowledged. But, although it has played a useful role in enabling new medicines to reach prescribers and patients, throughout Europe, much more quickly than was previously the case, it does have its critics and its successes need to be evaluated carefully.

EMEA – productivity, value and results

While EMEA is able to point to key statistics (see Table 4.2) showing it has been very busy since its establishment in 1995 (EMEA, 1999b) Kamran Abbasi and Andrew Herxheimer reported, in a BMJ editorial in October 1998, that:

> A recent analysis of European public assessment reports by the International Society of Drugs Bulletins, whose members are concerned with disseminating information about new drugs and drug safety to doctors, has echoed worries that the agency's standards of critical appraisal may be less rigorous than they should be.
>
> (Abbasi and Herxheimer, 1998; p. 898).

Table 4.2   Key figures on the work of the European Agency for the Evaluation of Medicinal Products, 1995–99: medicines for human use and mutual recognition procedures for medicines for human use

Total applications	195
CPMP Opinions*+	119
Community marketing authorisations granted	104
Variations to Community marketing authorisations	516
Scientific advice	104
Mutual recognition procedures completed	452
Arbitrations on variation applications	4
Variations to national marketing authorisations completed	1416
Arbitrations on variation to applications	6

Source: EMEA Status Report, London 25 May 1999b.
*Relating to 90 substances plus includes 3 negative opinions.

It should be pointed out, however, that Abbasi and Herxheimer go on to acknowledge that:

> in publishing public assessment reports, the EMEA is far ahead of most national licensing authorities – which are still notoriously secretive . . . indeed, the agency's continuing dialogue with the International Society of Drug Bulletins and national licensing bodies is likely to produce a more rigorous system,
>
> (Abbassi and Herxheimer, 1998; p. 898).

The speed with which events unfold, after EMEA has authorised a product, is also something that needs to be examined with a critical eye. Jean-Francois Dehecq, in a presentation to the Third European Round Table on the SEM in pharmaceuticals, brought forward disturbing evidence suggesting that there were lengthy hold ups in new medicines becoming available in some EU member states, even though EMEA authorisations had been given. Dehecq drew attention to the requirements of the EEC Transparency Directive, issued in 1989, which required that there should be no more than 180 days between market authorisation and market launch. The Directive also required that, in each member state, there should be published and transparent methods for pricing pharmaceuticals and an open and effective system to resolve disputes about getting medicines to market. He claimed that despite EMEA's hard work, supported by a Directive which had been in force well before its establishment: 'Outside Germany and Great Britain, where marketing delays remain reasonable, matters in other member states are not really improving.' Dehecq reported that the results of a survey of products marketed between 1986 and 1998 put 'the shortest marketing delay, after the grant of marketing authorisation' at 'three months – doubtless in Germany and Great Britain – whereas the longest delay is almost four years' (EFPIA, 1998: 24–5).

The widespread failure to move, within the times required by an EEC Directive, which had been in force since 1989, was underlined by an AIDS sufferer who made a presentation of his own to the Third Round Table. Colin Webb, of the European Network of Positive People, explained that he had been diagnosed HIV (Human Immunodeficiency Virus) positive in 1993. He had little doubt that his life had been greatly extended by new drug combinations that, to his horror, were not available to other EU citizens. Webb confirmed Dehecq's data on delays in moving from authorisation to market launch: 'Evidence shows', he said, 'that patients in certain member states can face delays (in getting access) to innovative medicines. On average medicines are first available in the last EU member state four years after the first!' (EFPIA, 1998: 26).

Fernand Sauer responded to Colin Webb's personal story and the comparative data for medicine launches by proposing that 'the one hundred or so companies' that had 'benefited from a European marketing authorisation should tell' EMEA 'in the coming weeks the story of their product in each country' (EFPIA, 1998: 30). EMEA subsequently held its third annual EMEA audit in London, devoting a significant amount of time to delays in getting approved products to market (EMEA, 1999c). It has also devoted considerable energy to improving its relationships with the many different public and social security authorities that have to meet the bill for new medicines throughout the EU. But the goal of speedy and uniform introduction of new medicines remains elusive (EMEA, 1999d).

Regulation and supranational bodies

The various roles and responsibilities of EMEA, the ECJ and the European Commission, in regulating access to pharmaceutical markets in the EU, raise important and interesting issues. How should the regulatory activities of supranational bodies and agencies themselves be regulated? What strategies should agencies, like EMEA, pursue to achieve the objects for which they have been established? To what extent should such bodies seek to influence public policy agendas – are they servants, collaborators or masters? To what extent should the legal principles underpinning European Law and ECJ decisions on trade in medicines be permitted to become key determinants in the formulation of health policies? Giadomenico Majone has studied these issues closely and written extensively about regulatory growth in the EU – considering both its causes and its effects (Majone, 1996: 263–77; 1998: 14–35). Majone has been able to draw on a growing academic literature about the dynamics of regulatory systems that operate with varying degrees of independence from nation states. There are, alongside the literature on the regulatory state, a growing number of publications about the involvement of the ECJ in regulatory issues, including health and health related cases (Taylor, 1997; Kuper, 1998: 39–58).

The institutions of the EU (the European Commission in particular) are said to be ill-suited to many of the activities we associate with a modern nation state. The principle of subsidiarity, for example, requires the Commission to leave as much as possible to member states themselves. However strongly European policy-makers may feel about economic inequality they are most unlikely to gain control of social security or taxation systems in member states. Although a number of member states have collaborated in the establishment of a European Central Bank the European Commission's role in economic policy making is negligible and likely to remain so. It has been suggested that the EU and its Commission can best be compared with the United States and its federal government in the late 19th and early 20th centuries. The EU has developed and is likely to go on developing primarily as a regulatory state. The early American state was 'a minimal state, a state of "parties and judges" with a highly developed party democracy that presumed the absence of a strong arm of national administration' (Richardson, 1996: 264). The EU, with its ECJ, that makes law for the EU as a whole, and its Commission, with strictly limited resources and powers, has only a few instruments of power, compared with those available to member states, to make and implement public policy.

The comparison, between the US, at the beginning of the 20th Century, and the EU, has been taken a stage further by Majone. He suggests that declining support for Keynesian economics, in late 20th century Europe, prepared the way for political leaders and officials to accept and adopt a role for public authorities focused on complementing and enhancing markets, rather than challenging or correcting them. However, even where markets are considered to be generally beneficial, there is support for public action to keep them honest and competitive. Support, in other words, for an umpire or regulator. Successful umpires are generally considered to be knowledgeable as well as fair. Umpires or regulators dealing with powerful rival interests – such as those concerned with the production, sale and use of pharmaceuticals – need to be well equipped to hold the ring. Regulators need to be able to find out what is really going on – when things are going wrong. They also need the independence and legal authority, to act decisively when things have gone wrong. The successful regulatory state is a state that can protect the public from defective and dangerous goods, root out dishonest practices and act against restrictive trading practices.

Majone provides a plenitude of evidence to support his view that the EU has been developing as a regulatory state. His evidence consists of details of the accelerating and substantial role of European institutions in formulating and introducing legislation, Directives and Regulations that apply throughout the EU. Noting, as he does so, that it was Jacques Delors, the former President of the European Commission, who predicted that by the end of the 20th century '80 per cent of economic and social legislation applicable in member states would be of European origin . . .' (Richardson, 1996: 265). A great deal of European regulation, Majone goes on to suggest, results from the determination of member states, often the member states that complain most bitterly about over-regulation, to see that other member states play fair. The Commission, limited as its powers and resources undoubtedly are, is ready to oblige member states with proposals for more effective regulatory mechanisms. After all opportunities to enhance the Commission's status and to extend its competence are most likely to come from developing its work as a regulator rather than from any other quarter. What is more the Commission is in the best position to obtain additional resources to support its work when it can claim to be providing services that member states have agreed they need and cannot provide on their own. Those who want an independent regime for regulating the trade in pharmaceuticals or a common set of rules and procedures for testing the safety of medicines, for example, are obliged to fund the arrangements which they believe are necessary. Good umpires don't come cheap. A supranational authority, lacking its own independent sources of revenue, cannot offer to meet the cost of establishing and operating a regulatory regime.

It is tempting to ask why member states – particularly those insisting most strongly on respect for the principle of subsidiarity – accept the case for supranational regulatory bodies. Majone's explanation is that ceding authority to supranational bodies, such as European agencies like EMEA, can have significant benefits and advantages for member states. Independent supranational institutions can serve to insulate national political leaders from domestic pressures and conflicts. Refusing to respond to pleas for action or additional funding, because they would be inconsistent with international obligations and the rulings of a supranational regulatory body, is much easier than simply rejecting them, because you disagree with them. Arrangements, that vest the authority for licensing medicines in a supranational body, can also help to build trust and confidence between member states. A supranational body, it is suggested, is in a better position to safeguard standards and agreements, between states and to weather shifts in public opinion or changes in economic circumstances and party control, than a body which depends upon a single member state government (Richardson, 1996: 268–9).

Giandomenico Majone's thesis about the origins of EU regulatory bodies and the growth of a European regulatory state is concerned with more than the motivation of political actors in member states. Majone is also interested in exploring the possible role of supranational regulatory authorities in formulating and implementing public policy and the consequences of developing and extending the European regulatory state. He quotes Terry Moe approvingly: 'Once an agency is created, the political world becomes a different place' (Moe, 1990: 143). Regulators can become powerful and independent in ways that their creators did not anticipate. Indeed that is precisely what he suggests has been happening in the EU. Specialists, with technical expertise, working in agencies that do not owe an unqualified loyalty to any single national authority 'are increasingly able to pursue their objective of greater autonomy . . .' (Richardson, 1996: 270).

Bodies such as EMEA and the European Agency for Safety and Health at Work, discussed in Chapter 2, present a considerable challenge to conventional political institutions. How should – how can – supranational regulators be regulated and made accountable? Majone's answer is that political accountability to elected representatives is unlikely to prove satisfactory. Elected representatives have neither the time nor detailed knowledge and motivation to pursue technical questions with the rigour that is required to hold specialist regulators to account. Rather, he argues that 'highly technical and discretionary activities, such as regulation' need to take 'self-policing' as their starting point. Majone observes that:

> US experience shows that regulators can be monitored and kept politically accountable only by a combination of control instruments: clearly defined statutory objectives, procedural constraints . . . judicial review, professional standards, monitoring by interest groups, even inter-agency rivalry'

> (Richardson, 1996: 274).

There can be little doubt that the autonomy and integrity of EMEA and its developing role in pharmaco-economics and pharmacovigilance will be a central feature of the European health policies of the future.

The European regulatory state includes the ECJ. In December 1996 the ECJ ruled on Merck *v* Primecrown (ECJ, 1996). Instead of ruling the so-called parallel trade in ethical drugs unlawful the Court determined that the free movement of goods could not be qualified, even in the case of medicines which were subject to price controls in individual member states. A price for a medicine, established in one member state, could be the price at which that drug could be purchased for resale anywhere in the EU.

Merck argued that companies at the forefront of pharmaceutical research, which were being paid different amounts in different parts of the EU for their products, were being treated unfairly. Parallel traders were making money simply by buying at a low regulated price in one country and selling on to another. The Court suggested that pharmaceutical companies could refuse to sell a patented drug in a member state where they thought there was a risk from parallel trading. David Taylor, commenting on the Court's advice in May 1997, described it as 'impractical (and) ethically offensive' (Taylor, 1997). The Court took the view that the implications, for health policy in the EU, were a matter for the Commission, the Council and member states themselves.

The Court's ruling serves to emphasise the dilemmas that confront regulators generally and regulators of the pharmaceutical industry in particular. How is it possible to know what is in the best interests of the public in general and the sick in particular? Measures which reduce the costs of medicines should, all other things being equal, mean that medical care system resources can be made to go further. But all other things are not equal. If pharmaceutical companies refuse to sell medicines because they consider that the prices they are being offered are too low then patients may be deprived of medicines or they may be prescribed less suitable medicines. If drug companies sell medicines at prices below those that are needed to fund research and a competitive pharmaceutical industry then Europe could lose out to the industry in America and Japan. The rate of innovation in Europe could fall along with employment and research activity. The ECJ was simply applying a fundamental principle of European Law. Merck and other pharmaceutical manufacturers were seeking to safeguard the future of their industry and exclude pharmaceutical traders who made money without adding value. The major purchasers of medicines in some of the EU's poorest member states were simply seeking to ensure that their limited health care budget went further. It is clear that there is no simple or universally acceptable way of reconciling a SEM, in pharmaceuticals, with improved access to pharmaceuticals in every part of the EU. In this area of European health policy it is far from clear who, if anyone, is on the side of the Angels. The Commission has a great array of possible partners but no easy or painless way to choose between them or to balance their interests.

5
The EU and Public Health

A public health department without parallel

The EU has a health department like no other. The European Commission's Directorate General V (DGV) Directorate F (Public Health and Safety at Work) has combined the roles of an international health promotion agency, public health directorate and health and safety policy co-ordinator, with those of a clearing house and commissioner for health research and policy innovation. To date health has not had a European Commissioner solely to itself or been allowed to assume the title EU Department for Public Health. Although the integration of Health with Consumer Affairs, in the Autumn of 1999, undoubtedly reflects the rising status of health in the Commission. Putting Consumer Affairs together with Health has meant, however, that public health, the health and safety at work and the health-related social insurance activities of the Commission are now to be found in separate Commission Directorates.

The Commission has no direct responsibility for the management of medical services. And it continues to encounter considerable opposition, from member states, at the merest hint that it might play a part in harmonising laws and regulations to do with health in member states (Belcher, 1997a: 2).

The combination of responsibilities and the strict limitations on its work reflect the surprising and serendipitous evolution of the EC's involvement in combating major health scourges and threats as well as the severe limitations on Commission competence outside these areas. The human form of 'mad cow disease', new variant CJD (nvCJD), which is discussed extensively in the next chapter, has put the policy boundaries between the Commission and member state health authorities under strain and under scrutiny. But, as this chapter will show, the involvement

of the Commission in health issues remains very deliberately circum-
scribed. This is so despite a reformulation of the EU's competence in the
public health field, following ratification of the Treaty of Amsterdam (in
1999). This Treaty contains a significant reworking of the EU's public
health aims and legal competence, which features in a discussion of the
future of the EU public health role towards the end of this chapter.

Before Maastricht – preparing the ground

It was the Maastricht Treaty, which came into force in November 1993, that
committed the EU to developing EU-wide policies aimed at improving the
health of all the EU's citizens. Before Maastricht and before the insertion of
Article 129 (the Public Health article), into a European Treaty, the EC and its
institutions lacked any specific authority to make or implement policies
which had the improvement or protection of public health as their
principal or sole justification. The SEA made it possible to piggy-back health
considerations onto the development of the single market.

Article 100A(3), which amended earlier European Treaties, required the
European Commission to advance the functioning of the internal market
by basing its proposals on the attainment of 'a high level of . . . health,
safety, environmental and consumer protection' (it now appears as Article
95 of the Consolidated Treaties of the EU). Thus, while the EC did not
completely ignore public-health issues, they were clearly a secondary
rather than a primary consideration (apart from those established roles,
considered and reviewed in earlier chapters). However, this was not
allowed to prevent the Commission seizing on opportunities, as they
arose, to move on to ground that went beyond any specific legal authority
that it possessed. It seems that there was a desire in the Commission to
promote the idea that European institutions had a role to play in
promoting the health of European citizens for its own sake. The
Commission and European political leaders who supported a bigger
health role recognised that they had no alternative but to adopt an
opportunistic strategy to public health. This opportunistic approach is
reflected in the development of the EC/EU public-health competence.
Indeed some might prefer to substitute the word haphazard for
serendipitous, used at the beginning of this chapter.

Europe against cancer

In three areas of general public health concern the Commission relied
upon liberal interpretations of general powers available under the Treaty

of Rome (HoC, 1992: 180). European campaigns were formulated and launched to deal with cancers, AIDS and drug dependency. The first of these, known as *Europe against Cancer*, dating back to 1987, is the most widely recognised and longest running special EC/EU public health programme. Chris Ham, in his account of the origins of EC involvement with public health issues, reports that 'Europe against Cancer . . . is believed to have originated through the interest of President Mitterrand' (Harrison with Bruscini, 1992: 138). It appears that the long-standing illness of this major European leader provided an opportunity for establishing a *de-facto* community competence. It seems probable that it would otherwise have been resisted by political leaders, most especially the British Prime Minister of the day, who were deeply suspicious of any Commission attempts to get a bigger slice of the action.

The first cancer programme, in the form of an action plan, was intended to run from 1987–89. It was targeted at well-known carcinogens and behaviours associated with the risk of malignant disease (CEC, 1993c). It promoted the European code against cancer, which embodies a good deal of common sense advice about how to live your life in a way that minimises risks associated with exposure to sunlight and an unbalanced diet. The first action plan sought to popularise the 'ten point code against cancer' (Box 5.1) – and had a fair degree of success in doing so. Despite its extraordinarily ambitious aim, to reduce cancer mortality by 15 per cent by the year 2000, the first *Europe against Cancer* programme, which contained 75 actions covering prevention, information and health education, as well as training for health workers and support for research, was judged by the Commission to have been a great success. The positive response to the programme, which the Commission has described as an 'original and significant' way of 'extending its action beyond the traditional action to combat carcinogenic chemical substances and ionising radiation . . . through new measures', was hailed as having lead to 'results [which were] on the whole very satisfying' (SCADPLUS). Whatever else can be said the first action plan, *Europe against Cancer*, was popular and inexpensive. The second *Europe against Cancer* action programme was drawn up to run from 1990–94 (CEC, 1990) and had, judging by the enthusiastic support for a third plan (approved to run from 1996 to 2000), succeeded in securing a permanent place for preventive work in the Commission and EU policy-making. Member state Ministers of Health, meeting in May 1993, decided to increase EU spending on the *Europe against Cancer* programme at the same time as they invited the Commission to present its proposals for a third action programme to combat cancer.

Box 5.1   European Code against cancer

Committee of Cancer Experts:
'If the European Code were respected, there would be a significant reduction in the number of deaths from cancer in the Community; the decrease could be about 15% by the year 2000.'

CERTAIN CANCERS MAY BE AVOIDED:

1. *Do not smoke*
   Smokers, stop as quickly as possible and do not smoke in the presence of others
2. *Moderate your consumption of alcoholic drinks,*
   beers, wines or spirits
3. *Avoid excessive exposure to the sun*
4. *Follow health and safety instructions at work*
   concerning production, handling, or use of any substance which may cause cancer.
      Your general health will benefit from following two commandments which may also reduce the risk of some cancers:
5. *Frequently eat fresh fruit and vegetables and cereals with a high fibre content*
6. *Avoid becoming overweight*
   and limit your intake of fatty foods

MORE CANCERS WILL BE CURED
IF DETECTED EARLY

7. *See a doctor if you notice an unexplained change: appearance of a lump, a change in a mole or abnormal bleeding*
8. *See a doctor if you have persistent problems,*
   such as persistent cough, a persistent hoarseness, a change in bowel habits or an unexplained weight loss
      For women:
9. *Have a cervical smear regularly*
10. *Check your breasts regularly*
    and, if possible, undergo mammography at regular intervals above the age of 50

Source: Based on *European File*, September 1990 11–12/90, 7 (CEC, 1990): 7.

The Commission's second cancer plan sought to focus attenti.. success in raising awareness of risk behaviours and carcinogens amongst European citizens. It strongly promoted recognition and understanding of the steps individuals could take to reduce their personal vulnerability. It was aimed at getting Europeans to act confidently and appropriately, by quickly seeking medical help and advice, if a malignant growth was suspected. Women were urged to check their breasts, regularly (the tenth rule in the European Code); all citizens were urged to limit the risk of skin cancers, increased risk being blamed on lengthy and unprotected exposure to sunlight. Particular emphasis was placed on educational work, aimed at school children. European health information carried a strong anti-smoking message. And battling with the tobacco industry has in fact become something of a European health theme.

The European Cancer Week, normally arranged for October each year, typifies the EU's enthusiasm for events which raise awareness of health problems and risks at the same time as they spread the message that Europeans have common problems and, thanks to the EU, some shared means for tackling them. In one account of EU work against cancer, during the Cancer Week held in 1995, Commission information providers note that:

> The media pressure created during the week (172 million contacts with Europeans), underpinned by a whole host of events . . . had a major impact on EU citizens' knowledge of cancer prevention. By the end of the campaign, over 20 million more Europeans were convinced that cancer is preventable. In addition, the various risk factors (lack of fruit, vegetables and cereals in diet, fatty diet, excessive consumption of alcohol, lack of physical exercise, smoking) were better identified , ... The 1995 European Cancer Week also helped to raise the profile of Community action in the public health field because 24per cent of Europeans said that they had heard of the Week and that they knew of the European Code against Cancer.'

(SCADPLUS)

Objectives and actions for improving the public health

Having begun by underlining 'the advantages of launching a European programme against cancer', at a Council meeting in Milan in June 1985, a Council meeting, this time in Luxembourg (in March 1996), adopted its third action plan to combat cancer. The plan referred to four broad objectives and four kinds of action. It supported a large number of specific interventions and initiatives. The action plan's acceptance seemed to underwrite a general acceptance of the idea that an EU role in 'ensuring a high level of health protection' should embrace not only high sounding general objectives but quite specific and detailed, albeit carefully judged, actions, directly funded through the Commission. The action plan to combat cancer for the latter half of the 1990s was aimed at:

- preventing premature deaths due to cancer;
- reducing mortality and morbidity due to cancer;
- promoting the quality of life by improving the general health situation; and,
- promoting the general well-being of the population, particularly by minimising the economic and social consequences of cancer.

The plan required the Commission to play a major part in combating cancer right across the EU through:

- data collection and research;
- information and health education;
- early detection and screening;
- training, quality control and guarantees.

The Council agreed that quite specific and detailed European actions and initiatives were required to:

- establish common objectives;
- standardise and collect comparable and compatible data on health;
- develop and strengthen the European network of cancer registers;
- organise programmes for exchange of experiences and of health professionals;
- disseminate information about the most effective practices;
- create information networks;
- launch European-scale studies and disseminate results;
- support epidemiological studies;
- focus on prevention;
- implement pilot programmes and pilot projects;
- compile reports;
- monitor measures taken;
- monitor early detection and screening activities;

- exchange experiences of quality control, of early detection of cancer, of prevention and palliative methods;
- contribute to the selection of priorities in cancer research and transfer the results of basic research into clinical trials.

(OJ, 1996: 9–15)

It has to be recognised, of course, that the more the EU, in the form of the Commission, becomes involved in public-health issues, the more sensitive its role has become from the point of view of some member states.

Public health and member state sensitivities

Two obvious illustrations of the sensitivity of its work on cancers can be found in tensions that have arisen between the Commission and the UK Government. In one case about tobacco advertising controls and, in the other, the dissemination of findings from EU funded research, into the early detection and treatment of cancers in different parts of the EU.

The arguments for the Commission, the Council and the European Parliament to act more decisively to ban tobacco promotion and cut tobacco subsidies – even if that means clashing with one or more member states – have been put powerfully by the *Economic and Social Committee* (ESC). It has the job of advising the Council of Ministers on draft European legislation. In an Opinion, issued in September 1994, on the Commission action plan to combat cancer, the ESC observed that 'this is not the first time that the committee has had to lament the blatant contradiction between the anti-smoking campaign and community funding of tobacco producers' (ESC, 1994: para. 3.4.3; see also Townsend, 1991).

The 'Bernie Ecclestone affair' and the embarrassment of Tony Blair – the UK's PM – dramatised the special arrangements which permitted continued tobacco advertising at formula one Grand Prix events and snooker competitions (well into the 21st century). The Euro compromise appeared to be at odds with the clear commitment of DGV to deliver a ban on tobacco advertising at all sporting events in the EU (DGV, 1997a: 11).

The United Kingdom also has good reason to be concerned at the unfavourable light in which EU funded research, into the standards and effectiveness of cancer services in different parts of the EU, has cast British cancer care. In the early 1990s the medical editor of the *Independent* newspaper reported that:

> Delays in getting treatment, rather than treatment itself, may account for poor results for breast, lung, ovary and cervical cancer in women

and stomach and colon cancer in both sexes. The proportion of British patients with stomach cancer surviving five years after diagnosis is about half the European average'.

(Hall, 1995: 6)

A BBC review, of the work of a panel of cancer specialists, published in February 1999, declared that:

'Cancer patients in the UK are less likely to survive than their counterparts in other European countries and the US because less money is spent on treatments. . . . The UK was found to be one of Europe's worst countries for cancer survival and one of the lowest spending on cancer treatment'.

(BBC Online, 1999a).

While the European Commission is under strict instructions not to get involved in the health-care systems of member states, policy makers and political leaders, throughout the EU, are aware that unfavourable comparisons can quickly enter the public domain. Comparisons can serve to highlight less successful and poorly funded services and become sticks with which to beat those who are responsible for national health services.

However attractive and positive the role of information provider and co-ordinator may appear to be – to the Commission – and however strongly it is presented as neutral, so far as member state health care systems are concerned, information can very easily be transmuted into unwelcome criticism of member state medical care systems. Claims that the Commission exists – so far as health services are concerned – simply to improve the quality of information and facilitate its exchange are most unlikely to insulate it from the hostility of member state governments when they believe it has had a hand in their political embarrassment.

Europe against AIDS

Experience with the *Europe against Cancer* programme emboldened the European Commission and member-state health ministers to, respectively, propose and back *Europe against AIDS*. The Council decision to set up the programme was taken in June 1991. The first AIDS programme was designed to promote prevention and to emphasise the role of information and health education. In 1993 the Commission extolled the strengths of its AIDS programme and garnered the support of member-state health ministers to continue the programme on into 1994. The Commission was very keen to develop, as persuasively as it could, arguments which supported the view that AIDS was a communicable disease which could be tackled most effectively by collaborative actions. The Commission claimed to be proposing a collaboration which it was uniquely well placed to facilitate and promote. The Commission explained, in one of its Communications, that there 'would be added value from the Community undertaking actions, particularly through economies of scale' (CEC, 1994h: 5).

The idea of *added value*, as a justification for a significant EU and Commission role in public health, has subsequently been presented as a kind of touchstone for EU actions and policies. Given the importance attached to subsidiarity in health matters and the Commission's desire not to step on too many toes, the idea that the Commission can bring something special to the party – an additional ingredient which cannot come from anywhere else – is an especially attractive notion. If it can be presented convincingly, it can help overcome objections to extending and strengthening the EU competence in the public health field.

Information included in the Commission's 1994 proposal for the continuation of its AIDS programme underscored widespread fears about the rapid spread of AIDS and the links between AIDS and other communicable diseases (CEC, 1994h). The consensus on the need for Community action, which the Commission's 1994 Communication on AIDS and other communicable diseases reported, reflected widespread fears about the rate of increase in AIDS cases in the late 1980s and early 1990s. Commission figures showed just 86 people as suffering from AIDS in the EC area in 1982. By 1990 that had risen to 13,500 and the 1993 Commission Communication, on the *Framework* for action in the field of public health, reported a further sixfold increase in the number of EC citizens recorded as suffering from AIDS (CEC, 1993b: Para. 63). There were, EU health ministers were told, no precise figures for those who were HIV positive but WHO estimates put the numbers in the EC area at 500,000 and drew attention to the 'recent resurgence of tuberculosis, often associated with AIDS' (CEC, 1993b: paras 63 and 64).

Abel-Smith and his colleagues, in an appraisal of EU health policy and priorities published in 1995, argued that:

> Aids is of particular importance at a EU level because of its increasing incidence, the absence of a vaccine or a cure, the potential impact of increasing mobility on future incidence and the scope for prevention'.
> (Abel-Smith *et al.* 1995: 15)

While there were many programmes being developed by member states themselves the Health Ministers who made up the Council agreed that the EU could add value to member state actions by promoting collaboration in the fields of information, education, social support, counselling, monitoring of HIV infection and staff training.

The implementation of *Europe against Aids* did not proceed as smoothly as the Commission had hoped; its AIDS work depended primarily on getting support to projects which had been submitted to and approved by the Commission. Some eighty AIDS related projects were under way by the end of 1992; getting them up and running stretched the Commission's 'limited financial and personnel resources' (SCADPLUS; CEC, 1994h). The process of approving and allocating funds to large numbers of projects meant that many started late and overran their original time frame. Problems with the administration of projects, particularly the management of budgets, left the Commission vulnerable to criticisms about poor financial control. These were criticisms of a kind that contributed to the resignation of the entire Commission, early in 1999. Because of delays in getting AIDS projects up and running the Council and the European Parliament were required to agree to the extension of the AIDS action plan (OJ, 1995: 1–6).

Given the requirement that European public-health action plans are genuinely multi-national and that they garner comparative information, from across the EU, it is easy to understand why their administration presents considerable difficulties for the staff of the European Commission. Nevertheless the *Europe against AIDS* programme directed most of its resources, in the early years, to relatively small scale projects aimed at prevention, social support and counselling. The amount spent on 'informing and increasing the awareness of the public and certain target groups' was increased substantially after the initial launch of the programme. Indeed the *Europe against AIDS* action programme is said to have been designed to give increasing emphasis to initiatives aimed at those reaching sexual maturity: 'activities targeted at young people in the field of culture, communication and information' (CEC, 1994h). Other EU policies have been available to focus resources on research. The BIOMED programme, at the heart of the Community effort to research disease, has included a substantial amount of work on AIDS and other infectious diseases. When the second action programme to prevent AIDS and other communicable diseases (set to run from 1996 to 2000) was adopted in 1996 total expenditure was held below Ecu50 million over five years – considerably less than the sums being invested in the Biomedical and Health Research Programme of the EU (BIOMED). The Commission –

given the numbers of individual projects for which it was responsible and the modesty of the total funding available – argued that it had to concentrate on being a catalyst for change and development. In its 1999 work programme DGV/F claimed that the activities it supported would impact on four areas:

- surveillance and disease control;
- prevention of transmission;
- information, education and training;
- support for persons with HIV/AIDS.

Good quality monitoring presents problems

The Commission is required to continuously evaluate the AIDS programme and report the results to the Council and the European Parliament. However, high quality evaluations of large numbers of diverse and modestly funded projects are impractical and assessments of the value of its work on AIDS and other public health areas have generally left supporters and critics, alike, unsatisfied. A determination to make as much descriptive material available as possible about its work programmes and the aims of the activities it supports has, perhaps, been more important to the survival and development of the Commission's public health action programmes than detailed evaluations. Especially where evaluations may cost almost as much as the action programmes.

In getting its general public-health competence launched the Commission has left itself open to criticisms that it has been far more concerned with processes than results. Indeed there have been good practical arguments for DGV/F to concentrate on building networks and collaborations. The Commission has certainly been busily engaged in European networking, in an attempt to bed down its public-health role.

Combating drugs misuse

Community activities to combat AIDS are strongly linked to European policies intended to tackle substance abuse. Intravenous drug-users are widely recognised as a high-risk group. They are considered to be both a source of the spread of HIV infection and particularly vulnerable to HIV infection at the same time. This is because intravenous drug-users combine three risk characteristics. The risk of infection by (and transmission of) the HIV retrovirus is associated with those who have direct contact with contaminated blood. This is a reflection of the risks associated with shared used of injecting equipment. The risk of sexually acquired infection – because of the likelihood of risky sexual behaviour, associated with the need to fund drug dependence through prostitution and the risk of vertical transmission – mother to child transmission of HIV. The interrelationships between substance abuse and HIV have served to reinforce the case for European action to combat drug misuse in the EU. This then is the third area in which the need for a European public health dimension gained acceptance prior to the coming into force of the Public Health Article in the Maastricht Treaty (Article 129) at the end of 1993.

If ever there was a field in which the benefits and advantages of European collaboration and the need for it seem to be assured it is surely substance abuse and drug control. The common interest of member states in regulating access to, trade in and use of drugs relates not only to controlling the spread of AIDS among substance abusers – and their sexual partners – but also to finding ways of reconciling different drug control policies and legislation in different parts of the EU. An EU that claims to champion a single market and free movement of all its citizens has good reason to be concerned about a trade in illegal drugs. Drugs that are considered a threat to health and a prime factor in law breaking. However, what is judged to be criminal in one part of the EU is viewed as a life-choice, which citizens are capable of making for themselves, in another part of the EU.

European documents contain numerous assertions about the need to promote an integrated and consistent approach to combating the use of illegal drugs and to tackling the health and social problems that they are believed to create (CEC, 1994f; IGC, 1997; Commission PR, 1999c).

The same Council meeting which, in 1986, resolved to make cancer the focus of Community action also called upon the 'Member States to draw on their experience in the treatment and rehabilitation of drug addicts [It would be necessary to do this in order to collaborate and inform] teachers, parents, and young people about the risks related to drug addiction.' The Council asked for 'a report and recommendations on measures' to combat drugs which could be 'taken at Community level' (CEC, 1993b: Para. 37). But, in the words of Commissioner Anita Gradin (the Immigration, Home Affairs and Justice Commissioner in the Santer Commission), this remains an area in which the starting point for any action plan is 'that every individual Member State is responsible for the fight against drugs in its own territory . . . [and the] . . . ambition on the EU level is to support and co-ordinate certain efforts in areas where the EU can bring added value' (Commission PR, 1999c).

Establishing the European Monitoring Centre for Drugs and Drug Addiction (EMCDDA)

So far as drug misuse is concerned the European Commission's activities on the public health front have focused on demand reduction; one of three aspects of illegal drug control, identified in European plans to combat drugs published in the first half of the 1990s. (CEC, 1994e). The other two are *Action To Combat Illicit Trafficking* (or supply reduction) and *Action at the International Level*

So far as measures aimed at reducing substance abuse are concerned the Commission has emphasised the contribution it can make by improving education and raising the quality of information about substance misuse. As illegal drugs became increasingly associated, in the popular imagination, with youth culture, it also became apparent that one of the principal problems faced by policy-makers in member states was the poor quality and limited comparability of data on use of and the morbidity associated with substance abuse. An illegal trade is a considerable obstacle to obtaining accurate information.

President Mitterand – who seems to have played a vital role in this area as well as in relation to *Europe against Cancer* – has been credited with persuading the European Council and the Commission to establish a European Committee to Combat Drugs (CELAD) (Farrell, and Strong 1992). CELAD, proposed by Mitterand, was established in 1989. CELAD recommended the establishment of EMCDDA which came into being in 1994. It is based in Lisbon and has the task of providing the Commission, member state governments and appropriate European institutions with comparable data on substance abuse. It is charged with playing a leading role in developing networks; networks to fight drug misuse and embrace national drug information centres, specialised agencies and international bodies (Bainbridge and Teasdale, 1995: p. 195). In its 1998 Annual Report EMCDDA's Executive Director, Georges Estievenart, claimed that EMCDDA had become 'a centre of excellence for addiction information . . . [and] . . . increasingly active in improving the knowledge base for policy-makers, practitioners and research alike'. EMCDDA had, since its establishment, become an 'integral component of EU activity . . . [reflecting] . . . with increasing accuracy and clarity the drug situation in EU countries . . . [and] . . . providing a basis for initiating systematic research and evaluation carried out by the EU and beyond' (EMCDDA, 1998a: 4). EMCDAA has also accepted a role in reviewing EU action on illegal drugs – an activity which is, undoubtedly, sensitive and inherently politically hazardous.

The interconnectedness of health policy

Anti-drug misuse policy provides a prime example of the interconnectedness and spill over potential of health and health-related policy-making in the EU. It is this interconnectedness which often explains the reluctance of member-state governments to accept enhanced powers and responsibilities for the European Commission and its agencies. National governments cannot be sure where additional powers and responsibilities, for the Commission or the supra-national agencies it has spawned, may lead. Linkage also helps to explain the constant stream of new requests and proposals emerging from the Commission and the European Parliament for more collaborative and integrated policy-making. Just a few illustrations – and there are many possible – from the illicit drugs field can help to make the point. EMCDDA used its first Annual Report to point out that 'most countries [in the EU] have witnessed rising totals for offences against the drug laws' and 'drug users often form 30 to 40 per cent of the prison population' (EMCDDA 1996: 5). European co-operation on the drugs front, even when it is focused on the health and social reintegration of drugs offenders, cannot help but raise a great variety of questions about drug-law enforcement and penal policies. In doing so it opens up debate about opportunities for and the need for increased commonality in dealing with drug offenders and offences. The same EMCDDA Report noted that: '. . . of the ECU 27.9 million spent by the EU in 1995, on anti-drug actions, about half was being spent outside the EU'. EMCDDA followed this up, in its second annual report, by noting that Ecu30 million, of an expanded EU anti-drugs budget, had been allocated to Bolivia – to fund a 'crop eradication and substitution programme' (EMCDDA, 1997: 10). The anti-drugs policy of the EU could easily be described as an important component of its embryonic foreign policy.

In relation to a pressing EU-wide health concern about the spread of infectious diseases, EMCDDA, as part of its work on monitoring Europe's drug problems, collated and publicised a substantial body of data to show that hepatitis infections, linked to drug use, posed a very considerable risk. Whilst EMCDDA reported, in its second Annual Report, that the rate of HIV infection amongst drugs users had been falling the same could not be said about Hepatitis C infection rates. The spread of Hepatitis C is a major public health threat because Hepatitis C is 50–100 times more infectious than HIV. Infection with Hepatitis C can lead to chronic hepatitis and extensive liver damage and/or cancer (EMCDDA, 1997: 6). With an estimated half a million infected people in the EU the spread of Hepatitis C really is a matter of common concern to EU healthcare systems

(EMCDDA, 1997: 7). Good ideas about minimising and reducing the rate of spread of Hepatitis C could, if spread rapidly throughout the EU, prove highly advantageous in holding down medical service costs in member states.

Given its brief to collaborate with governments and agencies beyond the EU EMCDDA's activities have served to highlight policy linkages in other ways. EMCDDA, in a press release (EMCDDA PR, 1998b) on the work of the US–EU informal drug forum, quoted General Barry McCaffery, who had just completed an eight-day US drugs fact-finding tour of European cities, approvingly. The General was quoted as saying that: 'by the turn of the century we must replace ideology with science [in the development of drug prevention activities]' (EMCDDA PR, 1998b). With widespread controversy about drugs laws and the information provided to schoolchildren, as part of drugs education programmes carried on throughout the EU, it is hard to read such a statement as other than highly critical of national policy-making and national political leaders. It is interesting, therefore, to note that EMCDDA seeks to – and is expected to – integrate its work on anti-drugs actions throughout the EU, with efforts to promote best practice. It does in fact collaborate with drugs specialists across the EU through The European Information Network on Drugs and Drugs Addiction (REITOX). REITOX is described by EMCDDA as:

> The European Information Network on Drugs and Drug Addiction . . . [It] . . . consists of National Focal Points (NFPs) set up in the 15 EU Member States and the European Commission.

EMCDAA goes on to explain that:

> Most of the Focal Points are expert centres in their own right, but some are still developing structures and functions to suit emerging needs. The role of a Focal Point involve[s] co-ordinating its national information centres to meet the EMCDDA's requirements for a set of core data, annual National Reports on the drug situation in each Member State and a national information network.'
>
> (EMCDDAa)

EU policy, as described in its public health *Framework* (CEC, 1993b), is focused on demand reduction. EMCDDA itself has described school based educational programmes as being 'at the heart of prevention in all EU countries' (EMCDDA, 1997: 7). While educational programmes are a national concern EMCDDA's partners in REITOX all agree such programmes need to be well informed and well presented.

The similarities and parallels between EMCDDA's determination and success in developing a European-wide network of specialist agencies and professionals, to share information and collaborate with each other, and the approach of the EASHW, are striking. Once again increasing use is being made of leading edge IT resources to share information and spread key messages. What is also very striking – however – is the modesty of the budget provision for EU internal anti-drug activities. EMCDDA's 1999 budget was set at Euro 8 million (EMCDDAb).

Not a great deal of money to work with

Details of actual spending by the EU on all its internal anti-drug programmes, in 1997, serve to emphasise the need for the Commission and its officials to find ways of working that have the strong support and active involvement of member states and all its many other partners. In 1997 Ecu33.3 million was spent on drug related work inside the EU – external spending accounted for Ecu20.1 million. The biggest slice of the internal budget (55 per cent) went towards work aimed at the 'reintegration of drug addicts'. EMCDDA received 19 per cent of the budget; public health projects were allocated just under Ecu5 million. Support for co-operation among EU justice systems received 3 per cent; vocational training, youth education and research received 6 per cent and work to combat money laundering received 2 per cent (EMCDDA, 1998a: 91–93).

There is a certain irony – given what many believe have always been parsimonious EU public-health budgets and particularly modest provisions for internal anti-drugs actions – that, when the TEU clearly defined the public-health competence for the first time that had grown up in the EC, drugs dependence – which many do not regard as a health problem at all – was the only *major health scourge* mentioned by name. Assertions that something is very important, that it is a great European problem that needs to be taken very seriously by the EU as a whole, so that it can be tackled co-operatively, are, most assuredly, not the same thing as firm commitments to devote large sums of money to it or to pool sovereignty, in order to do something about it.

Article 129 (the TEU defines the EU's role)

Article 129 of the Treaty on EU, the Maastricht Treaty, provided a secure legal base for EC-wide health policy and confirmed the Community's role in anti-drugs, AIDS and anti-cancer programmes. Its wording (see Box 5.2) suggested a very greatly enhanced and expanded role for the EU and, most particularly for the Commission. An enhanced and expanded role that heavily qualified by the prohibition on the Commission attempting any 'harmonisation of the laws and regulations of Member States' (European Communities, 1997: Para. 129 – 4 i). A minimalist view, that the Public Health Article of the Maastricht Treaty was no more than a tidying up measure, can be found in the Department of Health's response to a House

---

Box 5.2   Article 129 of the Maastricht Treaty (TEU) – the public health article

1. The Community shall contribute towards ensuring a high level of human health protection by encouraging co-operation between Member States and, if necessary, lending support to their action.
   Community action shall be directed towards the prevention of diseases, in particular the major health scourges, including drug dependence, by promoting research into their causes and their transmission, as well as health information and education.
   Health protection requirements shall form a constituent part of the community's other policies.
2. Member States shall, in liaison with the Commission, coordinate among themselves their policies and programmes in the areas referred to in paragraph 1. The Commission may, in close contact with the Member States, take any useful initiative to promote such coordination.
3. The Community and the Member States shall foster cooperation with third countries and the competent international organisations in the sphere of public health.
4. In order to contribute to the achievement of the objective referred to in this Article, the Council:
   – acting in accordance with the procedure referred to in Article 189b, after consulting the Economic and Social Committee and the Committee of the Regions, shall adopt incentive measures, excluding any harmonisation of the laws and regulations of the Member States.
   – acting by a qualified majority on a proposal from the Commission, shall adopt recommendations.

Source: Treaty of Maastricht – TEU – EUROPA web site.

---

of Commons committee report on *The European Community and Health Policy*. The Department of Health declared:

> the public health article (A. 129)[avoids] references to the delivery of health care, which is the responsibility of Member States . . . [and] places Community action on health competence on a sounder legal footing.' (DoH, 1992, Para. 1.2).

The Commission itself had anticipated the coming into force of the Public Health Article in November 1993, preparing a Communication (CEC, 1993a), for publication in November 1993. The Commission argued not only for the maintenance and development of its existing activities and sponsorship of work on AIDS, cancer and drugs misuse but identified a range of other public health programmes and activities. These were all areas where the Commission, working on behalf of the EU, believed it could add value; believed that it could achieve things in the public-health field that member states could not achieve at all – or as well – working on their own.

Integrating health into all EU activities and policies

Article 129 not only encouraged the Commission to think about doing more, in terms of the development of individual public-health programmes, it also created an EU obligation to ensure that 'health protection requirements [formed] a constituent part of [all] the Community's other policies' (see Box 5.2).

This truly awe inspiring responsibility, was addressed by the Commission in a report to the Council, the European Parliament and the ESC on the integration of health protection requirements in Community policies (CEC, 1995a) published in May 1995. The responsibility was also underlined by Article 3(o) of the Maastricht Treaty. Article 3(o) set the Community the goal of making a contribution to the attainment of a high level of health protection in the EU (it has become Article 3(p) following the ratification of the Amsterdam Treaty).

The Commission itself argued that Article 3(o) ' . . . opened up for the first time the prospect of developing a fully consistent and planned Community approach to public health, which would integrate the various strands of action being taken in this area into a coherent overall strategy with established priorities and aims' (CEC, 1995a: ii).

The Commission's approach to incorporating such broadly defined and far reaching responsibilities into its work programmes reflected the fact it was expected to accommodate this task within existing resources. The Commission decided to:

- reinforce existing arrangements for inter-service consultation whenever a decision might have implications for public health;
- set up an Inter-Service Group on Health, to ensure exchange of information and internal co-ordination with regard to health and health protection; and,
- produce an annual report which would include information about the health implications of other policies.

(CEC, 1995a: iii).

Somewhat tongue in cheek the second Commission report on the integration of health protection requirements in Community policies observed that 'it is not always evident how best to integrate health requirements in a given policy area, or how and according to which criteria to judge success and failure'. The Commission's conclusion was that 'Work will have to continue to develop thinking on these areas' (CEC, 1996b). Theresa Coghlan, the Brussels based EU Liaison Officer of the British Medical Association, went right to the heart of the matter when she wrote in *Eurohealth*, in December 1996, that: 'Informal discussions . . . lead [me] to the conclusion that the Interservice Group does not yet provide a satisfactory means of ensuring a balance in policy objectives . . . [U]ntil public health is pushed further up the policy agenda . . . leading Directorates, notably those concerned with economic and Internal Market issues, will feel little obligation to take the requirement seriously' (Coghlan, 1996: 6).

The circumstances in which public-health concerns become ubiquitous and move up the EU policy agenda – perhaps attain the summit, even if they are not destined to remain there – are the focus of a subsequent chapter. Theresa Coghlan's opinion, offered in 1996, was that 'economic aspects of the Community, including the Internal Market [remain] far more important than social aspects including public-health'. Coghlan anticipated contemporary debate about the future of the EU's broad public health responsibilities, when she suggested that if public-health concerns were to carry greater weight, were to cease to be 'a minority issue', a 'new Directorate-General with responsibility for public-health' would need to be established. She suggested, in her review of public health policy-making in the Commission, that the best prospects for promoting public health issues lay in 'strengthening links . . . between the related policy areas of public health and consumer affairs..with DGXXIV

(Consumer Protection) being expanded to take in both areas' (Coghlan, 1996: 6–7). This is more-or-less what has happened.

The Health Council – that is the Council of Ministers made up of health ministers from member states – which met in June 1999, added to the impression that when it came to health issues member states wanted to try and have it both ways. To make a public display of being attentive to the need to integrate health requirements into all Community policies – while tightly constraining the scope of EU public-health work. The June 1999 Health Council regretted 'that the fourth annual report on the integration of health protection requirements in Community policies had not yet been transmitted'. It urged the Commission to 'produce its fourth report as a matter of urgency' (Council PR, 1999b: 11–12). Michael Hübel, of the Commission's public-health unit, had already made plain the difficulties that the Commission faced in getting health concerns properly integrated into all its other activities when he wrote:

> In its Third report on the integration of health protection requirements in Community policies, the Commission acknowledges that 'Implementing the relevant objective in Article 129 is fraught with uncertainties as to what constitutes a high level of health protection, and what is the best methodology to arrive at reliable conclusions . . . '.
> (Hübel, 1998: 28)

He went on to stress the three factors which the Commission had consistently identified as essential for making 'real and sustained progress' in integrating health into all the Commission's activities and EC policy-making work. The message for member states was blunt. Much greater political commitment was needed. Member states would have to provide sufficient resources, most particularly 'expert resources in the public health area to shadow key policy sectors effectively'. The Commission had to be equipped with the means to monitor the impact, on health, of EU policies.

A scare, about dioxin in foodstuffs produced in Belgium, in the months leading up to the June 1999 Health Council, had once again focussed public attention on the ubiquity and unpredictability of health issues. At all its meetings, since November 1996, the Council has received reports on Transmissable Spongiform Encephalopathies (TSEs). Nevertheless a number of the ministers present represented governments determined to hold the line against European Parliament proposals for raising EU public-health expenditure. The Health Council has a history of standing out against proposals from the Commission and the European Parliament for substantial increases in funding for DGV/F's public health work. The divided political personality which the EU continually exhibits, on the importance of integrating health into all its activities, has been under-scored by the amended Public Health Article (Article 152, effective since May 1999).

The Amsterdam public health article

The revised article is intended to govern the efforts of the Commission to integrate health into every area of its work. What is more the article (see Box 5.3) requires the EU not only to protect human health but also to do all that it can to improve it. A requirement that the EU has found hard to meet as the history of European subsidy to growing tobacco demonstrates. Continued Community agricultural support, for growing tobacco, has been the subject of strong criticism from Commissioner Padraig Flynn (News EU, 1996c: 39; 1997a: 43; 1998b), serving to highlight the contradictory character of the policy portfolio the EU continues to maintain.

Article 153

The Amsterdam Treaty also led to the inclusion of another wide-ranging Article, under Title XIV on Consumer Protection. Article 153 could prove a very powerful instrument for those – both inside and outside the Commission – who want to unite concerns about consumer safety with a roving concern for the health aspects of other Community policies and activities. But public expectations, catch-all Treaty Articles and the political and economic priorities of member states will prove terribly difficult to reconcile unless member states show a greater willingness to accept that the Commission and its agents should have greatly enhanced authority and increased resources.

But – how do we do it?

There is, of course, a very considerable obstacle, quite apart from the inconstancy and inconsistency of political commitments, to fully implementing Articles 152 and 153. Michael Hübel puts it very clearly: 'The challenge is to develop an assessment methodology which is flexible, comprehensive and easy to apply' (1998: 28). To identify health problems early and to act decisively you need to be confident about spotting them and understanding them. In the face of the inadequacy of its own

Box 5.3   Article 152 – the revised public health article following Amsterdam Treaty

1. A high level of human health protection shall be ensured in the definition and implementation of all EC policies and activities.

   EC action, which shall complement national policies, shall be directed towards improving public health, preventing human illness and diseases, and obviating sources of danger to human health. Such action shall cover the fight against the major health scourges, by promoting research into their causes, their transmission and prevention, as well as health information and education.

   The EC shall complement the Member States' action in reducing drugs-related health damage including, information and prevention.

2. The EC shall encourage co-operation between the Member States in the areas referred to in this Article and, if necessary, lend support to their action.

   Member States shall, in liaison with the Commission, co-ordinate among themselves their policies and programmes in the areas referred to in paragraph 1. The Commission may, in close contact with the Member States, take any useful initiative to promote such co-ordination.

3. The Community and Member States shall foster co-operation with third countries and the competent international organisations in the sphere of public health.

4. The Council, acting in accordance with the procedure referred to in Article 251 and after consulting the Economic and Social Committee and the Committee of the Regions, shall contribute to the achievement of the objectives referred to in this Article through adopting:

   (a) Measures setting high standards of quality and safety or organs and substances of human origin, blood and blood derivatives; these measures shall not prevent any Member State from maintaining or introducing more stringent protective measures;

   (b) by way of derogation from Article 37, measures in the veterinary and phytosanitary fields which have as their directive objective the protection of public health;

   (c) incentive measures designed to protect and improve human health, excluding any harmonisation of the laws and regulations of Member States.

   The Council, acting by qualified majority on a proposal from the Commission, may also adopt recommendations for the purposes set out in this Article.

Box 5.3 *continued*

5. EC action in the field of public health shall fully respect the responsibilities of the Member States for the organisation and delivery of health services and medical care. In particular, measures referred to in paragraph 4 (a) shall not affect national provisions on the donation of medical use of organs and blood.

Source: EC (1997) Consolidated Treaties incorporating changes made by the Treaty of Amsterdam signed on October 1997 which came into force on 1 May 1999.

Box 5.4 Article 153 (Title XIV – Consumer Protection) of the Amsterdam Treaty

1. In order to promote the interests of consumers and to ensure a high level of consumer protection, the EC shall contribute to protecting the health, safety and economic interests of consumers, as well as promoting their right to information, education and to organise themselves in order to safeguard their interests.
2. Consumer protection requirements shall be taken into account in defining and implementing other EC policies and activities.
3. The EC shall contribute to the attainment of the objectives referred to in paragraph 1 through:
   (a) Measures pursuant to Article 95 in the context of the completion of the internal market;
   (b) Measures which support, supplement and monitor the policy pursued by Member States.
4. The Council acting in accordance with the procedure referred to in Article 251 and after consulting the Economic and Social Committee, shall adopt the measures referred to in paragraph 3(b).
5. Measures adopted pursuant to paragraph 4 shall not prevent any Member State from maintaining or introducing more stringent protective measures. Such measures must be compatible with this Treaty. The Commission shall be notified of them.

(*Source:* EC (1997) Consolidated Treaties incorporating changes made by the Treaty of Amsterdam signed on October 1997 which came into force on 1 May 1999.

resources DGV's line has been, has had to be, that 'the responsibility for ensuring that . . . [the obligation to make health a constituent part of all Community policies] . . . lies first and foremost with the originating Commission service' (1998: 27). Because Article 152 makes it a Treaty obligation to ensure that a high level of health protection forms part of the *definition* and *implementation* of all Community policies and calls on the EU to direct Community action to improving health, the task of developing and introducing transparent methodologies – which can be applied in widely varying circumstances – throughout the Commission's work, is a particularly daunting one.

The Health Council, held in June 1999, considered that the Commission should in future 'follow a problem-oriented approach and focus on issues of imminent importance . . .' (Council PR, 1999b: 12). But, such an approach, focused on issues of 'imminent importance', does not augur well for the coherence or effectiveness of Union efforts to integrate health concerns into all its work.

If the Commission is to avoid simply being moved up and down the beach, by each passing storm, it will need to invest heavily in developing robust methodologies, which travel well. This is an essential requirement for evaluating and testing all Union policies in terms of their health impact. If it cannot invest directly in a skills base of its own (to assess the health impact of policies, current or planned), then it will need to follow the alternative partnership route and find able specialist allies throughout the member states. Partners who are sufficiently strongly motivated to collaborate in building up a common approach and a common evidence base for evaluating EU policy for its potential health impact. How the Commission finds those partners and keeps them on board is something that occupies the mind of Jacques Bury, Executive Director of the ASPHER.

Bury argues that an effective EU public-health policy must be more than an early warning system. He makes two recommendations. They have been labelled *independence* and *evidence* – and they are closely allied. He proposes a body, directly accountable to the President of the European Commission, made up of academic specialists and people drawn from consumers' and citizens' organisations. 'This special inter-directorate body' would, according to Bury's plan, be supported by a small Commission secretariat and be given the job of directing the health impact assessment work of the EU. The independence of the 'special inter-directorate body' is critical to its prospects of success. Bury rejects the idea that appointments to his proposed inter-directorate health body could be controlled by or in the gift of member state governments. This would, in his words, simply 'duplicate the representation of national interests'. Although he does not suggest it, the membership might be determined by the European Parliament. It would be a development that could help to move the Parliament from the periphery to the centre of the European political stage.

Bury's second recommendation is for the adoption of an evidence-based approach to the work of the special inter-directorate body. This evidence-based approach should rely on 'a network of scientists', commissioned, as appropriate, from the EU's many scientific communities and supported by an 'independent core secretariat'. Bury's contention is that the analytical capacity required to support rigorous health impact screening, across the vast range of subjects with which the Commission is concerned, does not exist, 'nor should [it] exist in the European Commission'. It is time to 'think not in terms of a physical building [or]a large group of civil servantswhat is required are experts with permanent links to the scientific community'. The Director of ASPHER wants the EU to base its health impact screening work on the best evidence available; evidence he believes can only come from those who follow:

> scientific rules of excellence . . . and not the administrative rule of avoidance of political mistakes. In other words . . . experts . . . independent from political interference. That is the price to pay for gaining the confidence of the population.
>
> (Bury, 1998: 6)

The strategy Bury proposes looks upon the information age we are entering as an opportunity for the EU to take the lead in establishing multinational research communities, focused on informing health and health-related policy-making. Such communities would have a commitment to scientific methodologies and to obtaining and using the best evidence available. Such communities would – he suggests – lie beyond the reach of member state governments or national economic interests. Bury assumes that an independent network of scientists and policy specialists, collaborating and using the best electronic means, would also be committed to making findings as widely and speedily available as possible; using electronic means to do so. The extensive use of telematics in health is a theme in a later chapter. It is not at all difficult to imagine the anxiety that proposals of this kind are capable of generating amongst national political leaders.

Progress in adopting specific public health programmes

The strains that already exist in the institutional and political relationships at the heart of European health policy-making are evident from studying the course of EU public-health programmes, since the publication of the Commission's 1993 *Communication on the Framework for Action in the Field of Public Health* (CEC, 1993b). *The Journal of European Social Policy (JESP)*, which contains a quarterly digest of EU policy developments, reported (1997: 259) that only four out of the eight public health programmes proposed in the *Framework* had been adopted by the beginning of 1997.

The four adopted programmes included the continuation of work on AIDS and other transmissible diseases, a further iteration of *Europe against Cancer* and a programme on the prevention of drugs dependence. The fourth adopted programme could also be said to have elements that antedated Article 129 of the Maastricht Treaty. It was an action programme intended to support health promotion, information, education and training in member states. Ministers of Education from member states, meeting within the Council (in November 1988), had resolved to 'strengthen health education in schools and, to this end, make teaching material available to those concerned [and] provide training for teachers from the disciplines most affected'. The Education Council's resolution was complemented by a Health Council Conclusion, agreed in November 1992. It affirmed that: 'The school plays a vital role in ensuring that young people adopt a healthy lifestyle' and went on to identify other areas where '. . . health education is also of prime importance, e.g. local communities, homes, hospitals and workplaces' (SCADPLUS).

The EU health-promotion programme was, according to the Health Council, to receive a budget of Ecu30 million over five years. But the Council's funding package was challenged by the European Parliament, it wanted a budget of Ecu35 million and a more ambitious programme (News EU, 1995b: 39). The difference of view on funding this programme is one of a large number of examples of the Council and the Parliament clashing over the Commission's public health proposals.

There is a procedure, known as the *co-decision procedure*, which requires the Council and the European Parliament to concert their efforts in responding to and arriving at a consensus about Commission proposals. In the event that the European Parliament and the Council cannot agree there are arrangements for *conciliation*. Conciliation has become a regular stage along the road to the adoption of public-health policies in the EU. In the case of the Community Action Programme on Health Promotion,

Information, Education and Training it was the Parliament's view that eventually prevailed.

Matti Rajala, as Head of DGV's Unit F/3, described the five-year Ecu35 million package as encouraging member states to 'pool their ideas and experiences'. He was, he explained, firmly committed to the proposition that the '. . . key to disseminating health promotion throughout Europe is exchanging know-how and demonstrating models of good practice' (1998: 14). Perhaps the strength of existing international partnerships in health promotion helped the Parliament's case to prevail. Rajala pointed to a partnership with the Council of Europe and the WHO, in which the Commission contributed to health promotion work in hundreds of schools in 37 different countries. It is clear, however, that in many other instances the Parliamentary view on public health proposals and programmes has not prevailed.

Slow progress with four programme proposals

The other four programmes, proposed in the *Framework*, were concerned with *Health Monitoring*, *Rare Diseases*, *Pollution-related Diseases* and *Accidents and Injuries*. The road travelled to the adoption of all four programmes has been long and bumpy.

The Council had resolved, on 27 May 1993, that 'improved collection, analysis and distribution of health data [was] essential'. The Commission strongly endorsed that view when it issued its *Framework* document in November 1993. However it wasn't until June 1994 that the Council 'indicated that the collection of health data should be accorded priority and invited the Commission to present relevant proposals' (Decision No. 1400/97/EC). The Commission's proposal, for a five-year health monitoring programme, was issued in October 1995 (CEC, 1995c) with a proposed budget of Ecu13.8 million. Discussion at the Health Council on the proposal first took place in May of 1996. The European Parliament was strongly critical of the proposed budget and called for an increase of almost 50 per cent (News EU, 1996a: 34–5). Danilo Poggiolini MEP, speaking at the European Parliament in Strasbourg, in October 1996, 'expressed his dissatisfaction with the Council of Ministers decision to scale down the Commission's proposal'. What Mr Poggiolini wanted was sufficient resources to create a European Public Health Observatory which would be capable of bringing about a harmonisation 'of methods for compiling data on public health' (News EU, 1996c: 40).

The disagreements between Parliament, Council and Commission necessitated use of the conciliation procedure. When the Health Council met again, in November 1996, it debated the Commission proposal for a second time. The Council agreed to instruct the Committee of Permanent Representatives (COREPER) – a body made up of Brussels-based ambassadors from member states – to continue work on the monitoring programme proposal, so that agreement could be achieved in advance of the next Health Council (Council PR, 1996b).

'On 16th April [1997] the European Parliament and the Council . . . reached a compromise . . . the Parliament accepting the amount initially proposed by the Council' for the health monitoring programme (JESP, 1997: 259). When the Health Council next met, on 5 June 1997, it formally adopted, without discussion, the Programme of Community action on health monitoring. However, work on the creation of a European epidemiological surveillance network, to support the control of communicable diseases in the EU, considered at the same Health Council, still had to be 'forwarded to the European Parliament for a second reading under the co-decision procedure'. This was a distinct – but related – proposal on which it had taken the Council some time to reach a 'compromise' (Council PR, 1997a). A reading of the Draft Work Programme for Community action on health monitoring (1998–99) suggests that work had barely begun a year later on building the three pillars of Community health monitoring. Lyndsay Mountford, author of *European Union Health Policy on the Eve of the Millennium* (for the European Parliament's Committee on Environment, Consumer Protection and Public Health), observed, in September 1998, that 'Health Monitoring programme . . . [had] just started' (Mountford, 1998a: ix Para. E.2). The three pillars of the monitoring programme, as originally presented, were described as:

- a system of Community health indicators;
- a Community wide network for the sharing and transferring of health data between member states; and,
- methods and tools for analysing health status, trends and determinants (to inform health policy).

(DGV, 1998b)

The construction of each pillar would be a task of Herculean proportions. A few million Euro each year, which is all that has been made available, might help to maintain an established monitoring system with the Commission acting as a kind of central clearing house and most of the work required being undertaken by member states themselves. Mr Poggiolini's criticisms seem to be more than justified. Mountford found that the EU had sought to establish a system for the interchange of data on health 'ahead of having identified the relevant data set and . . . the most cost-effective means of transferring it' (Mountford, 1998a: 20 para. 2.53).

The other three 'new' public health action programmes have also suffered from long delays reflecting disagreements between the Council and the Parliament as well as the lengthy policy-making process and the co-decision procedures introduced by the Maastricht Treaty. It was not until May and July of 1997, over three years after the publication of its *Framework* Communication on Public Health, that the Commission proposed the three 'new' action programmes it had identified in November 1993; action programmes on injury prevention (CEC, 1997e), rare diseases (CEC, 1997d) and pollution-related diseases (CEC, 1997f). All three Commission proposals referred to action programmes that were to be begin in 1999 and to run until 2003.

There was an apparently straightforward case presented for each of the proposed action programmes. Injuries were identified as the leading cause of death in the EU between ages 1 and 35 and an important cause of morbidity amongst older people. The programme was intended to generalise the best accident prevention techniques throughout the EU.

Rare diseases were defined as diseases so uncommon that special co-operative efforts were needed and justified to tackle them. The programme would, it was hoped, facilitate work on rare diseases across the EU because, without the Commission's involvement, it was unlikely that the critical mass required to assist and inform patients, health providers and researchers would be achieved. Disease caused by or contributed to by environmental pollutants seemed a particularly appropriate target for EU action. The third programme was aimed at reducing pollutants and limiting human exposure to them – as well as contributing to work on finding ways to mitigate the adverse effects of exposure to them. The programme was notable because it was based on a joint initiative between DGV and DGXI (Environment, Nuclear Safety and Civil Protection). It was intended to focus particularly strongly on respiratory diseases and allergies.

It wasn't until December 1997 that European ministers of Health, at the Health Council, reached political agreement on the rare diseases programme and it wasn't until April 1998 that the Health Council formally adopted a Decision on the rare diseases programme. The proposed budget was Ecu6.5 million but it awaited a Parliamentary view (which was unfavourable) given in May 1998. Disagreements between the Parliament and the Council meant that the programme was made the subject of the EU's conciliation procedure. The Conciliation Committee, made up of equal numbers of Council and European Parliament representatives, has the task of settling on an agreed joint text when disputes between the Council and the Parliament are referred to it (Nugent, 1994: 317). A joint text emerged resolving disagreements on the rare diseases programme on 4 February 1999. Commissioner Flynn told the Parliament, on 13 April 1999, in urging it to support the agreed text, that it represented 'a first step in the right direction' (Strasbourg, April 1999). A first step in implementing a programme originally recommended by the Commission in its public health *Framework* Communication (issued in November 1993). The action programmes on pollution-related diseases and injury prevention, when they came to the Health Council of December 1997, were both described as being 'at a preliminary stage' (Council PR, 1997b: 7). The pollution-related diseases programme was adopted by the Council in April 1998, but only by a qualified majority. The Dutch delegation voted against the action programme (which had been allocated just Ecu3.9 million). Once again the European Parliament and the Council found themselves at loggerheads about the programme (News EU, 1999b: 50). The pollution-related diseases programme was then considered as part of the same conciliation process that examined the rare diseases programme. The results of the conciliation process being recommended to the European Parliament in April 1999.

At least some of the differences of opinion about the proposed injuries action programme appear to have been settled in favour of the European Parliament. The Commission's Communication on reducing accidents and injuries had estimated that accidents cost an estimated Ecu6 billion; it had referred to 20 million victims of accidents each year (in the home and outside it) and 100,000 fatalities. With the Dutch once again distancing themselves from a proposed public health action programme – and considerable Parliamentary opposition to the original proposal – the Health Council accepted a 'revamped proposal' in November 1998 (News EU, 1999a: 39,41; Council PR, 1998b: 4). The revamped proposal accepted a Parliamentary amendment to incorporate the European Home and Leisure Accidents Surveillance System Programme (EHLASS) into the scheme. The change boosted the five-year budget from Ecu6.5 million to Ecu14 million.

The European Parliament and the Council finally jointly adopted the Community action programme on injury prevention, within the public health *Framework*, on 8th February 1999 (Decision No 372/99/EC). As *Eurohealth* has pointed out, neither the European Commission nor the European Parliament were 'entirely pleased' about the way in which the

Council had handled the resolution of differences over the injury prevention programme:

> The Commission argues that the procedure [employed by the Council] is too bureaucratic . . . the Commission also took issue with the fact that some of the amendments it originally tabled were left out by the Council.
>
> (News EU, 1999b: 50)

Having been awarded its public health competence, by treaty, the EU – its Parliament and its Commission and, most notably the Social Affairs Directorate – has been struggling to emerge from the shadow of the Council. The Commission and the Parliament have been trying to discover and articulate a European voice about health issues.

Health issues galore

DGV/F has it fingers in many more pies than have been described so far. A look at the items that have appeared on Health Council agendas helps to give an impression of the significance and range of the many other health issues for which the Commission accepts or is expected to accept some responsibility. There is, for example, the issue of blood safety and the self-sufficiency of blood supplies in the EC/EU. Considered by the Council in June 1995 it was the subject of Commission Communications in May 1993 and December 1994. So-called *orphan medicines*, medicines needed for the treatment of rare diseases that attract little commercial interest, have also been a concern. Orphan medicines were the subject of a Presidency memorandum, considered by the Health Council in June 1995 and again in November 1995 (and subsequently).

In November 1996 the Health Council considered the Presidency's conclusions on a European Health Card – a *European health passport*. The idea of introducing such a card, which would facilitate the free movement of citizens of member states, dates back to 1981 (News EU, 1996a: 35). The European Parliament had called on the Commission, early in 1996, to submit a proposal for a card that could contain medical data, including data on an individual's blood group and allergies. The card would also hold details of an individual's social insurance cover and specify the arrangements that would enable a health provider to obtain reimbursement for the costs of medical treatment, wherever it was received in the EU. The Council noted that: 'a number of legal, ethical, economic and technical difficulties remain to be addressed'. But it also considered the Presidency's view that 'electronic cards could be generally introduced'. And it noted the encouragement given, by the Presidency, to the Commission, to 'pilot projects on the application of an electronic card . . . in the health and social security fields' (Council PR, 1996b: 15).

The Health Council of November 1996 also 'approved a procedure to be followed for Community participation in [an EU–US Task Force]' (Council PR, 1996b: 5). The joint Task Force had had its first meeting in Rome in May 1996 and has since been 'responsible for establishing [an] effective early warning system and response network for communicable diseases'. In June 1999 the Social Affairs Comissioner, Padraig Flynn, reported to the Council on the fourth meeting of the Task Force, which had met in Washington earlier that year. The Task Force was reported to have established three working groups to support attempts to 'strengthen[. . . the] existing international co-operation machinery for the surveillance, prevention and control of communicable diseases' (Council PR, 1999a, b: 12).

In June, 1997 the Health Council itself called upon the Commission to 'place before the Council and the European Parliament a Communication concerning . . . (i) cross border co-operation involving human organs and tissues intended for medical use . . . (ii) co-operation with international organisations concerned with public health . . . [and] (iii) current practice in the Member States on the traceability of organs and tissues . . .' (Council PR, 1997a: 6). And, in December 1997, the Health Council debated a Commission Green Paper on 'the principles of food law in the Community'.

The Health Council held at the beginning of June 1998 found it could reach political agreement on a recommendation 'on the limitation of exposure of the general public to electromagnetic fields'. It also agreed a very detailed Resolution on antibiotic resistance, which incorporated 'a [proposed European] strategy against the microbial threat' (Council PR, 1999b: 6, 8).

The range of issues considered and the scope for possible European actions on health, signalled by this simple perusal of the matters placed before the Council, is very striking.

Reporting health in the EU

No mention has been made so far of one solid achievement, flowing directly from the adoption of Article 129. The production of annual reports on the state of health in the EC. The first annual report was published in 1995 (CEC, 1995b). The report was produced with the assistance of the WHO Regional Office for Europe. It dealt with just 12 EU states (excluding new EU members Sweden, Finland and Austria). The rationale for the report was clearly set out by its authors who wrote: 'health problems are tending to become more and more international in character . . . [and] similar across countries as well'. They considered that it was important and worthwhile to lay the foundations for 'common solutions and to increase the exchange of experience and expertise' (CEC, 1995a: 1). A second report (CEC, 1997c) was published in 1997 and is entitled *The State of Women's Health in the European Community*. It has been widely distributed and is on sale throughout the EU. The 133-page report is a substantial document which contains a considerable amount of information about 'relevant health determinants . . . [and] health issues for women at various ages' (CEC, 1997c: 5). A third report, perhaps it should be described as the third EU bi-annual report on the state of health in the EU, was held up. The Health Council accepted that the '[transmission of] a third report . . . dedicated to the health status of migrants, . . . [should be] postponed to a later stage', so that it could 'take account of the particular health situation of Kosovo refugees entering the Member States' (Council PR, 1999b: 13).

Is it all too much for the Commission to handle?

Expectations of the Commission and the staff who deal with public-health issues – who are called upon to take the lead in ensuring that health issues are well integrated into all the EU's other policies – are vast and unrealistic. They considerably outdistance the Commission's current resources and overload its organisation. Expectations are in striking contrast to the powers and resources that member states are prepared to vote the Commission.

The mismatch has frequently been highlighted in *Eurohealth* – the house journal for close observers of the EU's health competence. Michael Joffe made the point, in June 1996, that the EU's CAP provided an £800 million (Ecu1000 million) subsidy to the production of tobacco. Observing wryly, as he did so, that 'very little of [the subsidised tobacco] . . . would probably be grown otherwise' (Joffe, 1996: 22). Caroline Jackson, MEP, writing for *Eurohealth* in October 1995, observed that 'if we really want a European public health policy . . . we will have to be prepared to pay for it' (1995: 14). She did not mince her words:

'What good can we expect a health promotion programme to do for a community of 370 million people when its total budget is 30 MECU over 5 years? How much can the staff of DGV devoted to health policy do when they number a maximum of 50?

(Jackson, 1995: 14)

Doeke Eisma, the European Parliament's EPHCPC draftsman, for its 1999 EU health budget proposal, told *Eurohealth* that he found it 'disappointing that Parliament and Council accepted only a moderate increase in the health budget and [then] put part of the budget in reserve because of [doubts about its] legal base' (Eisma, 1999: 12). He went on to write that he did not believe that 'the EU takes . . . EU health policy seriously' because 'the total health budget from the EU is less than 5 per cent of the EU premiums paid for tobacco [more than 999 million Euro]'. Eisma was in no doubt that it was essential to review and upgrade EU health policy. A review of EU health policy is underway and, in particular, proposals for reforming the way in which the Commission meets its responsibilities have become the focus of an extensive debate in Strasbourg and Brussels and beyond. They are also the focus of the final part of this chapter.

Reforming and reorganising work on health at the Commission

In July 1998 a freelance health economist, living in Luxembourg and on special leave from the (UK) Department of Health, Lyndsay Mountford, began work on a study for the European Parliament's EPHCPC. Her task was to produce, no later than 15 September 1998, a report on the future of EU health policy. The 11 weeks, during which she 'consulted 55 public health specialists' and reviewed the five EU public health programmes, led to the production of a remarkable and forthright report, *European Union Health Policy on the Eve of the Millennium* (Mountford, 1998a). The report is hard-hitting and highly critical of DGV/F. It contains many interesting proposals for the reorganisation of the Commission's health and health-related activities and explores a variety of ways of focusing the Commission's work more sharply on the health issues which lie within its competence.

Getting the needle

The Mountford Report was commissioned as a background study for an EU Parliamentary Committee Public Hearing on Health Policy. The Hearing took place at the end of October 1998. A British MEP and

EPHCPC member, Clive Needle, was given the task of taking the Public Hearing into account when reporting on and making recommendations (to the European Parliament) about a Commission Communication (adopted in April 1998) on the future development of public health policy in the EC (CEC, 1998a).

The Commission itself acknowledged, in its 1998 Communication that 'in order to build on what has been achieved . . . a new public health policy [was] required' (CEC, 1998a: 18). It identified six reasons for fundamentally revising the Community public health strategy:

- experience had shown up drawbacks in the current approach;
- new developments in health systems and in health had made change necessary;
- the Commission had been asked by both the Council and the European Parliament to 'present proposals for a new public health policy able to respond to the new challenges';
- the Commission itself wanted health policy to have a higher priority;
- change was necessary in order to respond to the 'challenges posed by the EU enlargement process' and,
- revision of the public health treaty article would lead to a broadening and deepening of the Community's responsibilities for public health.
                                                          (CEC, 1998a: para. 1, 1)

Lyndsay Mountford, called in to inform the work of the European Parliament, certainly agreed that a long (though she was only given a few weeks) hard look at the public health work of the Commission was necessary. Her criticisms, however, amplified and extended the Commission's own self-critical appraisal of its public-health activities.

Mountford found it impossible to interview DGV/F officers responsible for running individual public-health action programmes. The Director of DGV/F only gave permission for interviews to take place when 'most DGV/F programme officers were on holiday and the Luxembourg-based phase of the study was practically complete' (Mountford, 1998a: Para. 1.15, 4). Mountford was also denied access to DGV/F 'internal documents', although when she asked for documents which should have been in the public domain DGV/F was unable to find them and supply copies to her. She came to the conclusion that 'DGV/F has no systematic information retrieval system . . . i.e. library' and was concerned to discover that 'basic health references and journals' were not available in the Directorate (paras 2.67 and 2.68, 23). Lyndsay Mountford was able to talk to acknowledged 'international experts in each of the subject areas represented in the EU programmes' and to leading players in bodies concerned with public health across the continent. She came away, from interviews and her review of public health programmes, convinced that 'EU-sponsored projects [include] . . . good examples of work which can be done most effectively at international level' (Mountford, 1998a: para. E.7, x). Work on cancer registries and substance abuse and support for communicable disease surveillance networks were accorded high praise but many EU-supported public health activities were said to suffer from a '. . . lack [of] strategic planning' and from not having been 'selected against . . . technical criteria of "international value-added"'. Rather, she considered, the Commission had used the 'number of collaborators' as a key test (Mountford, 1998a: E10 and E11, xi). She drew particular attention, in the chapter of her report dealing with the cost-effectiveness of existing programmes, to the views of two commentators. They had: 'noted the vested interests which EU policy can create and the importance of bringing some projects to an end which have clearly fulfilled or outlived their function' (Mountford, 1998a: para. 2.69, 24). One of the principal criticisms of much EU funded public health activity made by Lyndsay Mountford was that it was focused, quite inappropriately, on health education and health promotion. Activities which most of the health specialists she interviewed believed could and should have been left to member states. It is an argument that the Commission itself has accepted and Padraig Flynn, in a speech at the Public Hearing, appeared to accept many of Mountford's other criticisms of Commission public-health work:

> it is essential [*he explained*] that we . . . [target] our limited resources to particular areas. And those areas are where the Community can provide, what I call, real added value. Let's not lose our sense of direction by trying to tackle too many different issues or cover too many separate agendas, however important each of them may be . . . [W]e shouldn't assume that every single subject that looms large for an individual member state will automatically be a priority for the Community. Not only are the EU's powers under the Treaty and our resources limited. In some areas it is also doubtful that EU action can add value to what member states are doing. Let me give you an example. In our public health programmes, we have supported a number of information campaigns. We did so in response to a widespread feeling that transnational campaigns could make an impact in a way that national or regional campaigns could not. Our experience has shown, however, that there are severe limitations to

what can be achieved at European level. Messages that work in Paris are not necessarily right for Amsterdam. Methods developed for Sweden are unlikely to be of immediate relevance to the South of Italy – or dare I say – in the West of Ireland'.

(Commission PR, 1998: 1).

Lyndsay Mountford had concluded that all too often the form of public-health programmes was a product of their 'political insertion' into the Commission's work plans and that the Commission had adopted a play it safe approach to the way in which tasks were carried out. Her personal recommendations, for the future of EU public-health work, were as uncompromising as many of her judgements about how public-health programmes had been managed in the past.

She recognised an 'overall feeling that the existing public health architecture [of the Commission was] no longer adequate to the demands which are placed on it' (Mountford, 1998a: vii). Not only should the Commission be prepared to reorganise radically and move public health staff from Luxembourg to Brussels – where most of the big Commission hitters are located – it also needed to demonstrate a real determination to employ high quality specialist staff. It was essential to find 'visionary leadership in promoting the health agenda across the Commission' (Mountford, 1998a: 40). Mountford was deeply critical of a 'recruitment exercise currently being run by the Commission for qualified health personnel'. The recruitment exercise, she wrote, was characterised by, 'poor or non-existent job descriptions', 'minimal selection criteria' and 'scrutiny . . . based not on CV but on somewhat less relevant criteria (such as the correct submission of application papers)' (Mountford, 1998a: 42).

Despite the very favourable reception given by the European Parliament, in March 1999, to the Needle Report – which was strongly influenced by Lyndsay Mountford's investigation and analysis – and the Commission's own declaration, in May 1998, that it would 'present . . . [detailed] proposals [for the future of public health] . . . as soon as possible after the Treaty of Amsterdam comes into force' (CEC, 1998a: 11), the decision making processes, required to reorganise and refocus public health work in the Commission, seem likely to extend well into the 21st Century. The Prodi Commission decision to amalgamate part of DGV with the Consumer Protection Directorate (DGXXIV) is just the start of what promises to be a lengthy process.

Member states will no doubt exert influence through a High Level Panel on Health. The High Level Panel on Health – a Committee made up of senior officials from member state health ministries – met in Freiburg during Spring 1999. It was announced after its initial meeting that the Panel had established working groups to consider the future of public health (and other health issues). Further progress with the review of the EU public-health role depends on reports from the Panel's working groups.

The Needle Report itself, tabled on 24 February 1999, represents the considered view of the European Parliament's EPHCPC, on the future of public-health policy in the EC. It responds directly to the Commission's Communication on the future of its public health role and incorporates ideas and comments from the Public Hearing on Health. The Needle Report welcomed the Commission's proposal to give priority to three types of action:

- improving health and health-related information and analysis;
- creating a rapid reaction capacity to deal with health threats; and,
- tackling health determinants through health promotion and disease prevention.

(*EP Report*, 1999: 6).

But this endorsement of the Commission's priorities was qualified by the observation that the Public Hearing – held in October 1998 – had supported the view that 'the most critical factor for a successful Community health policy was the integration of public health protection measures into all EU policies, with sound, transparent methodologies . . .' (*EP Report*, 1999: 10).

The EPHCPC was insistent that there should be 'a single Health Commissioner and Directorate General' for health, with 'enhanced expertise' and that the Directorate should be located in Brussels 'forthwith' (*EP Report*, 1999: 13). In its 11 proposals for action the EPHCPC sought to avoid 'the danger of a "shopping list" of worthy targets which cannot be tackled in a meaningful way' (*EP Report*, 1999: 11). It recognised that the Commission was entitled to complain that it has often been 'charged with duties beyond its means while being criticised for delays' (*EP Report*, 1999: 12).

Taking a lead from Mr Poggiolini

On 9 March 1999 Mr Poggiolini was, once more, present at a European Parliament debate. This time he was able to declare that he found Mr Needle's report 'excellent and most welcome' and to describe it as 'probably the last major health policy issue on which Parliament expresses an opinion before the end of [the] parliamentary term'. A new Parliament and a new Commission have been handed on the responsibility for redeveloping the Union's role in health, now Articles 152 and 153 are in force.

The Commission's ability to react rapidly to health threats – as the Commission Communication recommends it should be able to – is very much in doubt. It is far from clear that member states will accept the loss of national self-determination such a rapid reaction ability seems certain to require. If 'tackling health determinants through health promotion and disease prevention' is interpreted to include tackling social exclusion in member states, through EU actions, this may also prove to be a highly politically charged responsibility. But the politics of European health policy will have to take account of ECJ decisions that constrain the ability of member states to opt out. As the Commission's Communication on the future of public health pointed out in April 1998:

> The Court of Justice has confirmed [in Case C-180/96R, UK v. Commission ECR 1996, I-3903] that the objective set for the Community in Article 3(o) [now 3(p)] of the Treaty to contribute to attaining a high level of human health protection applies to all areas of Community policy which have an impact on health.
>
> (CEC, 1998a: 7)

A role for the Commission – helping members states learn from one another

Respect for the principle of subsidiarity is built into Article 152 and it is often suggested that it will shackle the EU's ability to prosecute its responsibilities for health successfully. There are two responses to such a proposition. Even though, employing John Peterson and Elizabeth Bomberg's words, 'subsidiarity became a leitmotif of EU decision making after the political crisis over the Maastricht Treaty in the early 1990s . . . *the way [remains] open to increased "policy transfer"*' (1999: 57).

Governments can and do 'learn from each other' – good ideas stand a good prospect of winning out and being widely adopted in an interconnected world. The first strand of the Commission's revised public-health policy is about encouraging and facilitating the transfer of good ideas and the sharing of experience. It is also the case that the principle of subsidiarity can help to deploy useful warning markers, capable of keeping the Commission and its agents out of areas that hinder rather than help the advance of *new-public health* priorities. As Lyndsay Mountford's report explained, to the EPHCPC, '. . . members of the public health community . . . fear that if the EU were to extend its activities into health services, the public health/disease prevention/health promotion agenda would get squeezed out in much the same way that public health is often the poor relation of high technology medicine at national level' (1998a: Para. 3.31, 32).

There is good reason for the Commission to do its level best to steer clear of any direct role in medical-care systems in member-states. It has much more important work to do, work that it is better placed to do. The real political problem for member state health ministers and governments is not losing control of the day-to-day management of their medical-care systems. The real – and essentially political – threat to their power lies in finding that the ability to set the public policy agenda, without reference to what is going on elsewhere in the EU, is constantly being diminished and eroded. Diminished among other things by a Commission developing itself as a focal point for a pan-European process of health evaluation. The Commission has the potential to become a conduit for many of the best ideas and the most up-to-date information about balancing health against economic growth and all the other desirable ends that the citizens of 21st Century Europe may espy.

PART II

The European Union and Health

6
BSE, Health Policy and Risk in the EU

The pervasiveness of risk

The ingredients that contributed to the so-called 'mad cow crisis' (Ratzan,1998) are in plentiful supply. The crisis mixture, made from ingredients that included (i) a new and previously unsuspected threat to public health, (ii) sensational press and general media coverage of that threat and (iii) uncertainty about the scientific data and explanations for the threat, proved to be highly politically combustible. The political flammability of public health crises is generally increased when health risks and news leaks about threats to health, cannot be contained within national frontiers. When international political pressures are added to domestic ones – national rivalries and suspicions act as an accelerant to purely domestic ones.

nvCJD is one of what appears to be a growing number of food-related public-health threats that are proving extraordinarily difficult to evaluate and manage. The genetic engineering of food, the widespread use of antibiotics in farming and the introduction of new chemicals into the food chain, by accident or by design, can all be (are all being) presented as threats to human health and well-being. All these issues, for example, have received coverage in recent years, in *Consumer Voice*; a European Commission DGXXIV publication designed for general circulation. DGXXIV is the European Directorate General responsible for consumer affairs which the new European Commission, led by Mr Prodi, is recasting as the EU's Directorate of Health and Consumer Protection (*Independent*, 19 July 1999).

To food-related health threats we can add many other matters which raise general health concerns. Threats to human health and well-being are often to be found on the obverse face of recently minted 'therapeutic advances' or 'scientific breakthroughs'. Michio Kaku (1998) whose *Visions* includes a very substantial section on 'The Biomolecular Revolution' – in which he discusses possible new therapies that may spin off from the human genome project – acknowledges the many risks and uncertainties which partner opportunities for making medical advances (139–261). Study of and interest in the sustainability of humanity's relationship with planet earth is another vast and rapidly expanding field. One that seems endlessly capable of generating new health concerns that are extremely difficult to assess and manage (see Gore, 1992: 99–114; WHO, 1998b: 58–64; Jukes, 1999: 198–202). Something that does seem certain, however, is that attempts to contain interest in and concern about such matters are bound to fail in open societies. Attempting to keep the lid on such concerns and manage information released through the popular press is likely to prove counterproductive, as the BSE crisis has amply demonstrated. Full and speedy disclosure, of what is and is not known about possible health threats, using direct and more sophisticated means to communicate with the public, is now possible. A good case for directness and openness is not too difficult to make (Chamberlain,1998: 169–74). It is a case that some in the European Commission and the European Parliament recognise, accept and even champion (DGXXIVb).

The European Commission, urged on by the European Parliament and in response to the Parliament's fierce criticisms of the Commission's part in the BSE crisis, claimed to have been convinced that greater openness was essential and eminently practicable. Its experience with BSE apparently played the decisive role in persuading it to give a much higher priority to ensuring greater transparency in relation to food-related health risks (CHCHP, 1997: Paras 1.1–1.5.3, 1–9; Santer, 1997). As this chapter will show the British and the European responses to BSE (Bovine Spongiform Encephalopathy) have much to teach us about the management of public-health threats. As well as the risks, uncertainties and opportunities that inevitably go hand in hand with closer political union and the establishment of a single European market.

Policy disasters – why do they happen?

Wyn Grant has described the BSE crisis in Britain as a 'clear example of a policy disaster' (Grant, 1997: 342). The vulnerability of British society to such policy disasters, he argues, should not be attributed to misfortune or the conjunction of 'unrelated [policy] mistakes'. Grant believes that Britain's vulnerability to 'policy disasters' reflects a style of government relying heavily on 'a self-confident administrative élite lacking knowledge of the field in which they are operating'. An arrogant and somewhat distant élite that combines a reluctance to admit its blind spots with an equal reluctance to 'make use of the full range of outside expertise' actually available to it.

Many of the elements found in Grant's account of the systemic failures of British Government in responding to the BSE crisis, also appear in accounts of the response of the European Commission and the Council of Ministers to BSE. The European Parliament was able to focus on these failures when it investigated the threat that BSE represented to the health of European citizens and the ability of Europe's administrative and political institutions to respond to a continental (even global) threat to public health.

The BSE crisis scored highly on the political equivalent of the Richter scale – perhaps it should be called the Major scale, in recognition of the damage done to the British Prime Minister's administration following Mr Major's deep and very personal involvement in the crisis.

The political impact of BSE in Europe

The impact of BSE on European politics and political institutions was very considerable. A reflection of the deficiencies and shortcomings discovered in the Commission and the Council of Ministers, by a newly confident European Parliament. A reflection also of the ways in which information about BSE and nvCJD came into the public domain. The strength of the political shock-waves was signalled by the Commission President's admission, made before the European Parliament in February 1997 (in response to its damning report – on inadequacies of the Commission's role in the gestation of the BSE), that:

> The BSE crisis has been one of the most difficult I have ever faced in my long political career. When I appeared before the [EU Parliament's] committee of inquiry I said it had taught me a lesson in modesty and humility. . . . Mistakes and errors have been made, some by the Commission itself.
>
> (Santer – speech to EP Strasbourg 18 February 1997)

The aftershocks have also been considerable – although it is far from certain that member states are prepared to accept fundamental changes in EU institutions and institutional relationships. Changes which, some close to the Commission believe, are vital in order to strengthen the EU's ability to act decisively when it is faced with major health crises, as it undoubtedly will be, in the future.

Disappointment, at the unwillingness of member states to agree enhanced Commission powers which would equip it to respond rapidly, decisively and robustly, as well as more independently to health threats, was a core theme of the keynote speech delivered by former Social Affairs Commissioner, Padraig Flynn, at a conference in Potsdam in January 1999. Flynn was describing the future he aspired to for EU health policy (Commission PR, 1999d: 2–3; News EU, 1999b: 52).

Tracing BSE back to its origins

The first cases of BSE have been dated back to 1984 and 1985 (BBC online, 1998b). The vets, who first encountered Mad Cow Disease, were puzzled – they were confronted with a previously unknown and invariably fatal neurological disease in cattle. The Ministry of Agriculture Food and Fisheries (MAFF) accepted, in 1986, that there was a new encephalopathy affecting cattle, and that the disease was a member of a group of transmissable encephalopathies already known to occur in animals and humans. In particular BSE appeared to share a good deal in common with a condition in sheep known as scrapie – a spongiform encephalopathy first recorded in Britain in the 16th century. Scrapie was a disease that had never been considered to be transmissable to humans (DG XXIV, 1996: 4). By the end of 1987 nearly 500 cattle were known to have been affected by BSE and detailed studies were started to build up an understanding and more complete picture of the disease. The number of BSE cases rose dramatically each year to a point, in 1992/93, when more than 3,500 cases were being notified each month.

The British Government's response to the rapid acceleration in veterinary reports of the disease was to make BSE a notifiable disease (in 1988) and to place a ban on feeding ruminants feed produced from the carcasses of other ruminants, such as sheep. The Government also instigated a slaughter programme for cattle suspected of having BSE and – in 1989 – introduced a ban on certain bovine offal entering the human food chain. Abattoirs had to extract Specified Bovine Offal (SBO) and ensure its safe disposal. SBOs included the brains and spinal cords of cattle – which had to be separated from animals processed through the UK's slaughterhouses. When the brains of cattle, which had died from BSE, were sent for post-mortem vacuoles, fluid-filled cavities, were found. The cattle brains were discovered to have a spongy appearance, similar to the appearance of brains taken from scrapie infected sheep. Suspicion fell on manufactured feeds provided to young dairy cows in many parts of Britain

– feeds that included the ground-up remains of slaughtered animals, sheep among them.

What appeared to have happened had not been anticipated. An ovine encephalopathy had jumped species, from sheep to cattle, and given rise to a bovine encephalopathy. An obvious question for the agricultural authorities and Britain's Ministry for food, faced with such a view of transmission, was whether one species jump could be followed by another. It was a possibility that they found very hard to accept and MAFF's reluctance to countenance, in public at least, the possibility that British beef could transmit encephalopathies to humans is one of the principal concerns of the Phillips Judicial Inquiry set up at the end of December 1997. The Inquiry was asked to 'review the history of the emergence and identification of BSE and nvCJD in the UK, and the action taken in response to it up to 20 March, 1996' (Phillips Inquiry, 1998).

The Phillips Inquiry was originally due to report in 1999 – its work will not now be completed until some time in the year 2000. One media report has suggested that the weight of documentation collected and produced by the Inquiry team necessitated a visit from structural engineers, who were asked to consider whether the inquiry building could take the strain (BBC online, 1999h).

A puzzling disease

BSE is a very strange disease and its development and transmission are unlikely to be fully understood for some considerable time (indeed it may be a scientific puzzle that is never fully understood). TSEs (transmissible spongiform encephalopathies) have been recognised, quite apart from the threat that they represent to animals and humans, as a great scientific challenge and (possibly) the product of a very unusual disease agent – a prion (*proteinaceous infectious particle*) (BBC online, 1998c).

The Phillips Inquiry has established that Sir Donald Acheson, Chief Medical Officer (CMO) at the Department of Health (DoH) from 1983 to 1991, telephoned Sir Richard Southwood, Professor of Zoology and Pro-Vice-Chancellor of Oxford University, to discuss establishing a working party on BSE in April 1988. Shortly afterwards the Southwood Working Party was announced. The Southwood Working Party Report recommended the establishment of another committee in February 1989. That committee, the Tyrrell consultative committee on research, issued its report in June 1989. In 1990 Spongiform Encephalopathy Advisory Committee (SEAC) was set up to advise on public policy and research into BSE. One close observer of the handling of the BSE crisis, Tim Lang – a

Professor of Food Policy and former advisor to the European Commissioner for the Environment – has argued that until the establishment of SEAC and the appointment of Professor John Pattison, who became SEAC's chairman in 1995, 'membership of [Government scientific committees dealing with BSE] was drawn from too narrow a pool of expertise' (Lang, 1998: 81).

Stanley Prusiner, who won the Nobel prize for medicine for his work on prions, the infective agents which it is now widely believed cause scrapie, BSE and vCJD, has argued since 1982, that prions can alter the shape of proteins. What is said to be almost mysterious is the way in which prions do this – even thought they do not carry the genetic information previously thought to be essential for the spread of an infectious disease. A prion does not reproduce itself in the way that a virus does, it is thought to 'corrupt a perfectly normal protein, PrP, which usually sits on the external surface of brain cells'. The prion, which 'recruits rather than creates' is responsible for a build up of 'insoluble deposits . . . within cells, which . . . [are] no longer [able to] function properly and die' (BBC online, 1998c). The disease agent is said to be extraordinarily difficult to destroy: 'This prion possesses exceptional characteristics, such as resistance to heat, ultraviolet and ionising radiations and chemical disinfectants' (DGXXIV, 1996: 3). Despite the spreading conviction that vCJD (the terminology variant CJD has widely replaced nvCJD) is a prion disease Prusiner himself is said to be sceptical about the link between BSE and vCJD arguing that: 'I am not convinced as a scientist that the new variant CJD is caused by BSE in cattle.' (*Daily Telegraph*, 8 June, 1998).

The world's leading authority turned down

Professor Prusiner, who gave evidence in 1998 to the judicial inquiry into the BSE crisis, explained that he had been turned down repeatedly by the UK authorities for a research grant to pursue his work on prions. A decision which he described as a 'major mistake' and which he is reported to have said 'cost us six years'. *The Financial Times* account of Professor Prusiner's evidence to the Inquiry quotes him as saying that if his research had been funded, 'it might have made a big difference'. *The Financial Times* story goes on to point out that Professor Prusiner had told the Inquiry that two formal applications made in 1991 and a third formal approach made in 1996, to fund work on the risk BSE posed to humans, using transgenic mice, had all been rejected (*The Financial Times*, 8 June 1998). A report, of the same date, in the *Daily Telegraph* quotes Professor Prusiner as indicating that he had now found himself in favour with the

UK authorities: 'They approached me a month ago.' The scientist, who was awarded his Nobel prize for medicine in 1997, for his work on prions, had 'been called in by the [UK] Government to plan new research into mad cow disease after years of rejecting his offers to help' (*Daily Telegraph*, 8 June 1998).

Criticism of the policy-making and informing process

Lang's principal criticisms of the policy-making process are built upon the proposition that, while it may prove difficult for experts who are trusted by Government, who are professionally eminent and widely respected, to admit the limitations of their own expertise, it is essential that they operate in an environment where they are strongly encouraged do so. Where they are expected to justify and explain their views and recommendations to sceptics and to ordinary folk. This will not happen – Lang suggests – if the policy-making process excludes non-experts (along with experts who are known to be awkward and unwilling to accept establishment rules and codes of behaviour). Even though Lang welcomed the appointment of Professor John Pattison to SEAC he continues to castigate the political and policy-making establishment for its reluctance to 'include consumer and other representatives on key committees such as SEAC' (Lang, 1998: 81–2). The reluctance of the British Government to include such representatives is said to: 'lie . . . at the heart of the failure of Government since 1988 . . . SEAC should be widened to include consumer, environmental health and social science expertise'. SEAC's annual report for 1997–98 included a recommendation supporting the appointment of 'a representative of the public interest' (1998: Para. 9, 7). Professor Sir John Pattison, whose role Lang had welcomed, gave up the Chairmanship of SEAC in June 1999, following his acceptance of the post of Director of Research and Development at the Department of Health.

The BSE epidemic in cattle did lead to heightened surveillance of CJD – the spongiform encephalopathy known to occur 'in man throughout the world at low levels' (NAO, 1998: 96). From May 1990 the National CJD Surveillance Unit at the Western General Hospital in Edinburgh maintained a special alert for any signs that the occurrence of CJD was increasing or changing. By spring of 1996 the Unit at the Edinburgh hospital had 'identified 10 out of 207 cases [reported to it] since 1990 [as having] features which distinguished them from other cases . . . [The 10 cases] had come to the Unit's attention between March 1995 and March 1996' (NAO, 1998, 96).

SEAC, led by Professor Pattison, wrote to Stephen Dorrell, the Secretary of State for Health, and Douglas Hogg, the Agriculture Secretary, in December 1995, about the transmissability of spongiform encephalopathies (Phillips Inquiry – timeline). On 20 March 1996 SEAC announced that 'the CJD Surveillance Unit had identified a previously unrecognised and consistent disease pattern' and concluded that 'the most likely explanation is that these [CJD cases] are linked to exposure to BSE before the introduction of [the ban on Specified Bovine Offal introduced by the Government] in 1989' (Phillips Inquiry – timeline). On the same day the Agriculture and Health Ministers made statements to the House of Commons. Subsequently a series of Government Orders were issued which prohibited the sale for human consumption of any meat from bovine animals over 30 months old and provided for their slaughter and the safe disposal of their carcasses.

Alarm at what was happening was not limited to the UK public. The European Commission issued a Decision (96/293, 27 March 1996) that prohibited the UK from exporting live cattle, their semen or embryos or the meat of bovine animals slaughtered in the UK. The EU prohibition on UK beef exports extended to any bovine materials liable to be consumed by other animals or by humans and materials used to make medicines and cosmetics. The previously very limited European controls on UK beef exports, in operation between 1990 and 1996, themselves became the focus of severe European Parliamentary criticism. The criticism was directed at the British Government and the European Commission, as well as the Council of Ministers. While the comprehensive and open-ended European beef ban became the focus of British Government anger with the EU and its Commission they were presented, in the UK, as a justification for a British campaign designed to frustrate EU decision making (Grant, 1997: 347).

The European Parliament takes centre stage

The European Parliament was able to take the centre of the stage. It made use of its Rules of Procedure to investigate the circumstances in which Britain has been permitted, largely unconstrained by Treaty obligations and European regulations or the veterinary inspection work of the European Commission, to carry on with an international trade in beef and beef products. It was also able to investigate a highly suspect trade in animal feeds – thought to be the source of BSE and of its spread. In the course of July 1996, during the European Parliamentary sitting, MEPs decided to establish a temporary committee of inquiry into BSE. The

Committee started its work in September 1996 and adopted a report in February 1997, which was highly critical of the Commission and the British Government.

The Medina Report, named after the temporary committee's Rapporteur, Mr Medina Ortega, is a deeply disturbing document. The Committee found that 'the main evidence of mismanagement of the BSE crisis [could] be traced to the period 1990/1994 . . . 75 per cent of the cases of BSE recorded in the UK occurred between 1990 and 1994' (*EP Report*, 1997a: Para. 1.C). Instead of public health and animal health considerations driving the work of the Commission the majority of Medina committee members concluded that commercial and trade considerations had been uppermost in the minds of senior figures in the Commission and that they had allowed themselves to be bullied by UK officials. Members of the Medina committee were convinced that the British Government had behaved improperly and thereby limited Commission action to investigate and act on the dramatic increase in BSE affected livestock in the UK. The evidence that the committee collected in the course of its investigation was hard won and often obtained, in the committee's opinion, despite the obstructive and unhelpful attitude of the British Government and the European Commission itself (*EP Report*, 1997a: Para. 1.B). The Commission was accused, for example, of employing 'blocking tactics [and] concealing the truth on various sensitive issues', while the British Minister for Agriculture 'refused to appear before the Committee of Inquiry'. The British Government was found to have 'adopted blocking tactics'; the committee concluded that this 'meant that a number of [their] questions remained unanswered'. The Committee found that 'BSE stemmed from the introduction, into Europe, from the United States of the "Carver-Greenfield" system of manufacturing meat-and-bone meal'. The British Government, unlike the governments of other member states, had accepted the imported process without insisting on an 'adequate sterilisation period' (*EP Report*, 1997a, Para. 2). The European parliamentarians noted that the UK Government had ignored the advice of one of its own Royal Commissions, which had reported in 1979 and had questioned 'the wisdom, from an epidemiological point of view, of feeding rendered animal remains to ruminants' (*EP Report*, 1997a: Para. 2.1.b).

The European Parliamentary committee was convinced that the British authorities could and should have acted earlier and acted more decisively. The possibility of BSE jumping from one species to another, from cows to humans, was – the Medina committee argued – recognised as early as 1988. When, in December 1988, the UK authorities 'prohibited the use of milk from suspect cattle for any purpose other than that of cows feeding their own calves', they were acknowledging that there 'was a risk to public health if people ate meat from animals affected by BSE' (EP Report, 1997a: Para. 2.1.c). So far as the European Parliament's inquirers were concerned the failure of the British authorities, to pursue concerns about the possibility of BSE spreading to the human population more vigorously, was compounded by the UK Government's inaction in controlling the sale and export of potentially contaminated 'feedingstuffs'. When the Committee of Inquiry asked Sir Richard Southwood, who had been in charge of the UK Government's Working Party on BSE, what he would have advised the UK Government to do, if he had been asked about the use of existing stocks of meat-and-bone meal in 1988, he replied:

> if you ask me whether in 1988 the working party would have considered there was a risk to herds in other countries if UK-produced meal (with meat-and-bone) was exported I am totally confident that we would have answered in the affirmative. Knowing that the meal was almost certainly the cause of the outbreak in the UK it is clear that it was irresponsible (whatever the law) to make it available as cattle food elsewhere.
>
> (*EP Report*, 1997a: Para. 2.2.c)

The Committee discovered when they examined data supplied by Mr Packer, Permanent Secretary at MAFF that, 'just after the ban [in 1989] on feeding meat-based meal to ruminants in the UK, exports to the EU rose to 25,005 tonnes (as opposed to 12,533 in 1988)'. They were understandably disturbed that:

> UK animal feed producers continued to export their product to third countries (exports to the EU doubled after the ban in 1989) in spite of the then alleged links to BSE and unclear labelling of the origin of the ingredients.
>
> (*EP Report*, 1997a: Para. 2.3)

A distrust of the UK and its controls on exports was sown – a distrust that is proving hard for the British authorities to overcome.

The Committee's investigation of the relationship between the UK and the European Commission's specialist committees and inspectors gave rise to even more anxiety about the behaviour of the British Government and the way in which the Commission had failed to meet its responsibilities, to EU citizens, for food safety. Mr Hoelgaard, a senior Commission agricultural directorate official, the key Directorate official with responsibility for veterinary issues, told the Committee that:

At the end of an inspection discussion . . . with UK veterinary services on 29 June 1990 when BSE was raised by the [European] inspectors . . . Mr. Keith Meldrum, Chief UK Veterinary Officer, apparently reacted angrily, stating that *the Commission inspectors had no authority to investigate BSE matters . . . BSE was not a technical but a political matter . . . the UK provided the best certificates in the world* and *the Ministry of Agriculture was reluctant to install computers in abattoirs due to the issues of cost and confidentiality.*

(EP, 1997a: Para. 2.4 – author's emphasis added)

The Committee established that there had been no BSE-related inspections by European veterinary inspectors between 1990 and 1994. They went on, quite understandably, to 'deplore the fact that top-ranking officials in DG VI . . . bowed to the wishes of Mr. K. Meldrum . . . even though . . . [European] inspectors had [previously] uncovered BSE-related deficiencies in some [UK] slaughterhouses'. Mr Meldrum had, the Committee were told, informed colleagues at one meeting of the European Standing Veterinary Committee, that, while 'people were worried about this new disease', BSE was 'more an issue of consumer confidence than consumer protection'.

The 'preponderance of UK scientists and officials' at meetings of the Scientific Veterinary Committee – which advised both the European Commission and informed the work of European Standing Veterinary Committee – was another cause for concern for European parliamentarians investigating the background to the BSE crisis. The Committee of Inquiry determined that 'the UK was able to control [the Scientific Veterinary Committee] through the convening of the meetings, the agendas and attendance, and the drafting of minutes' (*EP Report*, 1997a: Para. 3.2). The Standing Veterinary Committee gave advice to the Council of Ministers – on the basis of specialist advice it received from the Scientific Committee. The European Parliament's Committee of Inquiry concluded that the role of UK nationals in the EU's Scientific Veterinary Committee led to a situation where the Veterinary Committee's recorded views reflected 'current thinking at the British Ministry of Agriculture, Fisheries and Food' (*EP Report*, 1997a: Para. 2.5). The Committee of Inquiry also noted that some members of the Southwood Committee had 'said publicly that minutes of its meetings [Southwood Working Party meetings] were drawn up by a UK Ministry of Agriculture official and [contained] omissions and discrepancies' (*EP Report*, 1997a: Para. 2.6).

The European Parliament's Committee of Inquiry was convinced that attempts to improperly influence the work of the Commission and the

Council could also be found at the most senior levels of government. They discovered that, when seeking to get the Commission and the Council to modify restrictions on the export of gelatin, the then British Prime Minister, John Major, had written to the President of the European Commission personally. Mr. Major wanted to make sure that Jacques Santer appreciated the 'imperative need for the ban on gelatin, tallow and semen to be fully lifted'. Mr Major was said to have informed the President that Britain would be putting its 'full weight into persuading other Member States' (*EP Report*, 1997a: Para. 2.10). The President of the Commission told the European Parliamentary Committee of Inquiry that 'he regarded the attitude of the British Government as a form of blackmail'.

When, in May 1996, the Scientific Veterinary Committee recommended lifting the ban on gelatine, tallow and semen and the Standing Veterinary Committee voted against it, John Major is said to have regarded the Standing Committee's decision 'as a breach of faith'. The decision to launch 'Britain's policy of non-co-operation with the EU' has been attributed to his anger with the decision (Grant, 1997: 349). Mr Major had earlier signalled his attitude towards the Commission when, faced with an EU Commission 'beef ban' he rang Jacques Santer to complain. *The Financial Times* reported that, 'in 10 incandescent minutes [John Major] . . . distilled his frustration and bitterness . . . towards Europe in its struggle to contain the crisis over mad cow disease' (Parker, B. *et al.*, 1996; Southey, 1996). President Santer himself later described his 'first phone contact with Mr Major . . . to discuss the problem [as] . . . "rather an argument" . . . Mr Major . . . had "threatened legal action"' (*The Financial Times*, 16 January 1997).

The British Government did indeed begin a legal action against the Commission. An action that has come to have an important place in European health policy and will almost certainly become more important still in the years ahead. The same *FT* news story noted that the President of the European Commission had confirmed accusations and suggestions that the UK had used '"threats and blackmail" in its attempts to get the global ban on British beef exports lifted'.

The personal politics of BSE

John Major's very personal involvement in the management of the BSE crisis and the UK's negotiations with the Commission about its beef ban have been highlighted in a story entitled 'Hogg: Major ignored me on BSE'. The story appeared in the *Independent on Sunday* in 1998

(22 November) – after the Phillips Judicial Inquiry into the BSE crisis had been established. The former Conservative agriculture minister was said to have 'warned John Major that Britain was facing a "national calamity" when scientists established a link between "mad cow" disease and its human form CJD'. Mr. Hogg wrote, as Agriculture Secretary, to the 'Prime Minister and other members of the Cabinet . . . [but] his appeal for the . . . government to set up a judicial inquiry was ignored'. Mr Major has recently confirmed his personal determination to resist a total ban on beef products in March 1996. He made his decision against the advice of his Agriculture Secretary (*The Financial Times,* 7 May 1999). As the *Independent on Sunday* anticipated members of the former Conservative administration had become involved in a 'vicious blame game', in the course of appearances before the Phillips Judicial Inquiry into the handling of the BSE crisis in the UK.

European Parliamentary criticism of the European Commission

The Medina Report was not only critical of the British Government it was strongly critical of the European Commission. It found that the division of public health responsibilities among Commission Directorates and the compartmentalisation of the Commission's health and consumer protection work had 'hampered the co-ordination and efficiency of the services concerned [and] facilitated the shifting or responsibility for maladministration between the various services of the Commission'. The compartmentalisation of Commssion activities had made a bad situation worse because the Directorate responsible for agriculture (DG VI) had arrogated 'primary management of BSE to itself' (*EP Report,* 1997a: Para. 3.4). Just as in Britain, where parliamentarians were critical of the failure to face up to the conflicts of interest European parliamentarians were critical of the Commission's failure to separate consumer protection work from the administration and regulation of Union agriculture and agricultural support policies. The Committee also found that the principle of subsidiarity had been presented as an excuse for 'errors such as the failure on the part of the Council or the Commission to implement or monitor Community law' (*EP Report,* 1997a: Para. 4.3). The European Parliament temporary committee concluded that failures in the Commission and the Council meant that national interests and commercial interests had repeatedly been considered ahead of public-health protection (*EP Report,* 1997b).

Some of the Medina Reports strongest criticisms were directed at former Agriculture Commissioner MacSharry. Mr MacSharry is represented as having repeatedly frustrated efforts to ensure that there was a full and open discussion of BSE in the Council of Ministers during the early 1990s. Mr McSharry's attitude both alarmed and appalled members of the European Parliamentary Committee of Inquiry. In June 1990 Mr MacSharry made 'public threats to take out infringement proceedings against Member States' which wanted to place restrictions on British beef exports. He was said to have made no attempt 'to commence infringement proceedings against the UK for failure to comply with its [EU Treaty] obligations . . .' over BSE related matters. In September 1990 Mr MacSharry was reported to have issued an instruction to Mr Legras, the Commission Director General for Agriculture, to stop any meeting on BSE taking place. When Mr MacSharry appeared before the European Parliamentary Committee on 19 November 1996, to give his evidence and answer questions, he 'failed to answer repeated and quite explicit questions' about the 'suspension of all BSE-related checks in the UK between 1990 and 1994'. The Committee came to the conclusion that the Commissioner had either ordered the suspension of the checks or turned a blind eye to their suspension (*EP Report*, 1997a: Para. 4.1).

The Committee declared in its report to the European Parliament:

> That the Commission's handling of the BSE affair has been lacking in transparency is obvious from the contradictions existing in the ex-Commissioners' and the DG VI officials testimonies and in the numerous pieces of written evidence which have appeared in the press or been supplied by the Commission to the present committee.
>
> (*EP Report*, 1997a: Para. 4.2)

The Committee was in no doubt that, if the Commission had had a properly organised and independent machinery for multi-disciplinary advisory committees on public-health-related issues, it would have stood a much better chance of making 'a correct assessment of the evolution of the [BSE] epidemic and the possible public health risks' (*EP Report*, 1997a: Para 4.7).

The President promises fundamental reform of the Commission

When Jacques Santer came before the European Parliament in Strasbourg on 18 February 1997 to respond to the Medina Report and the Parliamentary debate about it he was confronted by a considerable body of European Parliamentarians who wanted to formally censure the Commission for what they considered to be its mishandling of the BSE crisis. The text of his speech to the Parliament includes admissions of responsibility and promises of reform.

Jacques Santer acknowledged 'mistakes and errors' and the need to 'learn the lessons of [the] crisis and bring in reforms to make [the] Union more democratic and safe' (Santer, 1997: Para. 15, 7). The President promised that the Commission would act to 'rectify the shortcomings . . . described in the [Medina] report' (Santer, 1997: Para. 8, 3). Changes were needed and would be introduced to:

- the Commission's administrative structure;
- the system for scientific consultation;
- the decision-making machinery;
- inspection methods; and,
- the Community legal bases for action.

Jacques Santer announced that in future:

- responsibility for legislation would be separate from scientific consultation;
- there would be rigorous selection of the best scientists (with guarantees of independence);
- no barriers between the work of different expert committees;
- responsibility for legislation would be separate from that for inspection;
- there would be greater transparency and more widely-available information throughout the decision-making process and inspection measures;
- dissemination of the opinions of scientific committees would include the creation of a public database on the internet;
- acceptance of the need to consider and disseminate minority scientific opinions.

The President told the Parliament that he looked to European parliamentarians to help in the fight for the resources and staff to ensure that the Commission could do its work properly on behalf of EU citizens. He had, he said, been particularly impressed by a report to the French National Assembly. Mr Mattéi had, in his report to the French National Assembly, concluded that:

> The people involved are less to blame for the breakdowns in the system than are the contradictions of the system itself, *which does not make full allowance for the effects of a single European market on public health.*
> (Santer, 1997: Para. 12, 5 – author's emphasis added)

Jacques Santer, aware of the UK Government's action in the ECJ – to overturn the 'beef ban', told the Parliament that the EU needed the legal authority to act decisively in response to public health threats. He promised that the Commission would be doing its best to 'persuade the Member States . . . that legislative decisions [on the CAP and agricultural production] should be taken by the co-decision procedure.' (Santer, 1997: Para. 14, 6). A procedure that requires the involvement of the European Parliament in the European policy-making process. The Parliament should, he argued, be more deeply involved in future and the Commission was determined to make much more use of Article 100a of the EC Treaty, which provided for the approximation of laws between Member States, rather than Article 43, found under the Treaty's agriculture title. This would make three things possible:

- improved co-ordination of Member State policies;
- harmonisation, where necessary, at the Community level in the field of human health; and,
- co-decision on health-related matters.

In a final flourish Santer claimed that it was his belief that 'the time has come to put health to the fore in Europe' (Santer, 1997: Para. 14, 7). In the event the legal basis for Commission action on food safety and agricultural matters has been advanced rather more strongly by the ECJ than by any changes agreed between member states to the legal base for EU agricultural policy-making (Roth-Behrendt, 1998: 3). Ironically John Major and his Government can count themselves among the principal architects and authors of that advance.

The British Government, the ECJ and health in the EU

Mr Major's threat to Jacques Santer to launch a legal action against the Commission 'beef ban' was borne out. On 24 May 1996 the UK Government brought 'an action under Article 173 of the EC Treaty for the annulment of the Commission decision 96/239/EC of 27 March 1996' (ECJ Judgement 5 May 1998: Para. 1). The British Government had also sought the immediate suspension of the Commission's 'beef ban' – while its legal action before the ECJ was being decided. The ECJ dismissed this application on 12 July 1996 (ECJ Press Release, 1997).

The UK Government case accused the Commission of exceeding its legal authority in introducing the 'beef ban' and disregarding EU law on the free movement of goods. The British Government went further and argued that the Commission had misused its powers and failed to give sound reasons for introducing the ban. It was suggested that the Commission was more concerned about influencing consumer opinion rather than the strength of the scientific case for a ban. The Commission's ban was, it claimed, disproportionate as well as unjustified and 'founded on an inappropriate legal basis . . . Article 43 of the EC Treaty' (ECJ, 1998: Para. 31). The UK Government's case disputed that there had been an outbreak of disease which constituted a 'serious hazard to animals or human health' covered by EU Directives. It also asserted that 'risk to human health . . . did not justify [the EU ban because] . . . it was negligible', given the control measures which had already been adopted (ECJ, 1998: Para. 32).

The European Commission for its part argued that its ban was entirely justified and consistent with European Treaties and European law. Its case was that SEAC's pronouncement in March 1996 about the existence of nvCJD and the likely origin of that new human disease, had fundamentally altered the situation and justified an immediate world-wide prohibition on the export of beef and beef products from the UK. A world-wide ban was appropriate, in order to exercise effective control over the re-importation of British beef into the EU. It was a ban that the Commission had legal authority to introduce.

The ECJ decisions to dismiss the UK Government's action and rule the UK case for annulling the Commission's ban inadmissible appear to have greatly strengthened the Commission's authority. There can be little doubt it has the legal authority to act rapidly to control trade when it has good reason to believe that the public health may be threatened. The ECJ's judgement declares that:

> the Commission's powers . . . are drafted in very wide terms, inasmuch as they authorise the Commission to adopt "the necessary measures" . . . without imposing any restrictions as to the temporal or territorial scope of those measures . . . [I]n the event of a zoonosis or disease, or any cause likely to constitute a serious hazard to animals or to humans, the immobilisation of the animals and/or products and their containment within a specific territory constitutes an appropriate measure . . . [I]t must be recalled that the Commission enjoys a wide measures of discretion, particularly as to the nature and extent of the measures which it adopts, the Community judicature must, when reviewing such measures, restrict itself to examining whether the exercise of such discretion is vitiated by manifest error or a misuse of powers. . . . In the present case, the publication of new scientific information had

established a probable link between a disease affecting cattle in the
United Kingdom and a fatal disease affecting humans for which no
known cure yet exists'.

(ECJ, 1998: paras 54–61)

The Court also took the view that it was necessary to apply common sense
guidelines to the requirement, laid upon the Commission by Treaty, to
provide reasons for its decisions. The ECJ has been firm in applying Article
190 (now Article 253 following the Amsterdam Treaty). The ECJ declared
that 'the degree of precision of the statement of the reasons for a decision
must be weighed against practical realities and the time and technical
facilities available for making the decision' (ECJ, 1998: Para. 70). The
Court went on to point out that:

'In the present case . . . the Commission gave as one of its reasons . . .
the SEAC announcements . . . [It made] reference to the adoption of
measures by the Member State with the greatest experience of BSE [the
UK] [This] constituted in itself a sufficient statement of reasons for the
decision by the Commission to likewise adopt additional measures'.

(ECJ, 1998: para. 71)

The ECJ appeared to accept that, while the Commission was entitled to
rely on Article 43, it might have been well advised to consider broadening
the legal base of its action and drawing on other EC Treaty Articles.
Articles giving it the authority to act decisively when it suspected that
there was a serious threat to public health and safety. In a striking passage
in its judgement against the UK Government, the Court referred to
Articles in the EC Treaty that required the EU to develop policies '[aimed]
at a high level of [human health] protection . . .'. The UK Government's
legal representatives were reminded that the EC Treaty committed
member states to the proposition that EU policy would be 'based in
particular on the principles that preventive action should be taken . . .
[and that] environmental protection requirements must be integrated
into the definition and implementation of other Community policies'
(ECJ, 1998: Para. 100).

Having failed comprehensively before the ECJ the United Kingdom was
ordered to meet the Commission's costs in the action. The UK suit before
the ECJ had resulted in a judgement that underlined and reinforced the
priority that the European Treaties accord to human and animal health. It
enhanced the Commission's authority to act decisively when it believed it
was entitled to do so. Articles 152 and 153 of the TEU, as amended at

Amsterdam in October 1997 and the aftershocks of the BSE crisis – among which the ECJ judgement against the UK judgement must be counted – have provided the Commission with a considerable amount of political and legal capital. The political machinations, the behind the scenes activities and conflicts that characterised the BSE crisis should, nevertheless, serve as a reminder of just how difficult it is likely to prove in practice to use that capital to advance the cause of European public health. Beyond the management of crises, European policy-making still hinges on agreements arrived at between member states in the Council of Ministers and at Intergovernmental Conferences (IGCs).

Health scares and public policy

David Davis undoubtedly had a point, when he described the 1980s and 1990s as 'the decades of the health scare' (Bate, 1999: vi). He found it paradoxical that, 'as people are remaining healthier and living longer than ever before', ill-founded or exaggerated health scares should attract more media attention than ever before. The paradox was all the greater because the risks and hazards associated with such things as smoking, alcohol consumption and the use of the private motor car don't generate anxieties in proportion to the threat to well-being they represent. Similarly there was an unbalanced perception of natural and manmade hazards. Natural environmental hazards, like radon gas, seemed to generate far less anxiety than industrial synthetics that become the focus of press attention.

Davis is surely entirely justified if he is taken to be suggesting that keeping risk in perspective and learning to live with uncertainty should be every bit as important as respecting the precautionary principle. Respect for the precautionary principle is what leads most of us to expect public decision-makers, confronted with new and poorly understood or evaluated risks, to behave with extreme caution. We all know and understand that respecting the precautionary principle can be expensive. We are also aware that expectations that the precautionary principle *must be respected* often rest on emotion rather than a detached assessment of the costs and benefits of watching and waiting to see what happens.

The BSE crisis illustrates the expense and the emotion that are an integral part of contemporary health-related food scares very well. In its report on the *cost of the crisis*, published in 1998, the National Audit Office informed the UK Parliament that:

> In 1996–97, expenditure on BSE-related schemes amounted to £1.5 billion . . . [NAO anticipated additional] expenditure of £1.9 billion . . . between 1997 and 2000. Between April 1996 and September 1997 [the schemes paid for] . . . the slaughter of 2.6 million animals . . . [A] trade worth some £520 million annually [was subject of the EU trade ban]'.
>
> (NAO, 1998: 1, 11)

The BBC has provided an even higher estimate for the value of the international trade in British beef lost following the EU ban, putting it at nearly £650 million a year. The BBC report on 'Britain' s bill for the mad cow crisis', made in June 1999, claimed that:

> No-one doubts that farmers were hit hardest. Cattle prices fell [and] farmers incomes plummeted from £4.1 billion in 1996 to about £1 billion in 1998. . . . One bank reckoned that 25,000 farmers were driven out [of business].
>
> (BBC online, 1999c).

The numbers of lives saved and the number of lives lost, because of the way in which the precautionary principle has been applied, will no doubt be disputed for many years to come. When the Department of Health published figures for deaths from vCJD up to May 1999, in July 1999, it reported that there had been 42 confirmed vCJD deaths in the UK.

The fact that emotion and science often pull even the most rational of individuals in different directions was underlined by Professor Prusiner's reply to a question put to him by one member of the Phillips Inquiry team. When the Professor interrupted a flight from San Francisco, to stop off in London to give evidence before the Phillips Inquiry on Saturday, 6 June 1998, he was asked whether he had changed his diet in any way since learning of BSE. Professor Prusiner replied:

> Let me be fair about this. I have worked in this field for 25 years. And before there was ever BSE I mainly worked on scrapie. . . . Did I go out and eat lamb chops, did I go out and eat lamb brain, sheep brain? The answer was "no", but it was not based on scientific criteria it was based just on emotion. It is what I said earlier. When there is a disease like BSE things do not sound very appetising. But at a scientific level, I cannot give you a scientific basis for choosing or not choosing beef, because we do not know the answers'.
>
> (Phillips Inquiry – daily transcript for 6th June 1998: 61–62).

BSE – one of many complex health-related issues for the Commission

BSE is just one of a growing number of complex health-related issues which are commercially and politically sensitive and which fall within the competence of the European Commission. There can be little doubt that many of them will end up coming, by one route or another, to the attention of the ECJ. Whether it is genetically modified food or insurance premium calculations, based on risk assessments that take account of an individuals genetic susceptibility to disease, health-related issues threaten public decision-makers with more and more political and legal minefields. They also confront policy-makers with the even more uncertain minefields of public opinion. Threats to health and safety often arouse strong public emotions and rate as exceptionally newsworthy, even when risks to the public are modest or negligible or simply impossible to quantify. As Peter Sandman has put it: 'Journalists are in the news business, not the education business or the health promotion business' (Sandman, 1999: 275–6). Health policy-makers and those who wish to influence them have little choice but to recognise that, as Sandman has put it, 'the mass media are in the outrage business'. Sandman's content analysis of the coverage of environmental risks on American TV nightly news bulletins, between 1984 and 1986, led him to conclude that it is: 'timeliness, proximity, prominence, human interest, drama, visual appeal, and the like' which determine coverage. '[C]overage', as Sandman explained, isn't primarily a reflection of risk, '. . . it is about blame, fear, anger and other non-technical issues' (Greenberg *et al.*, 1988; Sandman, 1999: 276). Sandman, however, does not 'blame' or hold the mass media responsible for creating outrage, he is convinced – and this is what he says he tells his corporate and government clients – that the mass media merely *amplify outrage* (Sandman, 1999: 276–7).

Fear and anger are powerful emotions that are constantly being fed and engaged by public perceptions of hazard and threat and blameworthiness. Fear and anger are emotions that help to fuel the processes, political, administrative and legal, which make change possible. But these most combustible of human emotions, to pursue the conflagratory imagery with which this chapter started, can burn with an alarming ferocity. They are only likely to be sustained for short periods of time. They may well burn up or burn out those who are fired with them and make little lasting difference to human behaviour, the law or to public policy.

European health policy-makers have, largely through the BSE crisis, learned just how flammable health threats can become and how they can exert a temporary and somewhat unpredictable influence on the politics of health. They have also learnt something about how European institutions can be shaped and policy priorities can be determined – at least for a while. They have yet to learn how to ride – to use quite outrageous imagery – health scandal tigers, confidently and successfully and avoid being consumed by them.

Considerable skill and determination will be need in future to direct and sustain the energy that is released by mounting concern about the impact that commerce, science and technology have on our food, our environment and, through them, on our health. The very busy Commission DGXXIV for *Health and Consumer Protection* has been sending out strong signals that it takes the health and the protection of European consumers very seriously indeed (CEC, 1997g, 1997h and 1998d). European citizens must surely wish the Directorate, with its expanded role in health policy, every good fortune in managing an extraordinary portfolio which can be relied upon to continually spring surprises.

7
Health, Information and the EU

Commission enthusiasm and member-state reluctance

The European Commission has, for some time now, been pursued by academics and health specialists who want it to play a major role in promoting and co-ordinating the effective use of information about health and health services in EU member-states (Abel-Smith *et al.*, 1995: 125–43; Belcher and Mossialos, 1997c). The Commission is undoubtedly attracted by the idea of becoming an important player and a partner for member-state health-care systems (Abel-Smith *et al.*, 1995: xi–xii), even if it is expressly forbidden, by Treaty, from seeking a direct role in managing or harmonising health services. A closer relationship with member-state health-care providers and health ministries would be very welcome to the Commission, it would affirm support for the EU's health competence and provide enhanced opportunities to develop it.

Relationships, falling short of matrimony, which bring together national bodies and supranational bodies, can be fruitful. A closer relationship between the Commission and member-state health-care systems is widely considered – by academic health-policy specialists (see Abel-Smith *et al.*, 1995; Ham, 1997; Saltman, 1997a, 1998; Mossialos and Le Grand, 1999, for examples of the academic literature promoting the idea of international collaboration) – to be essential if information systems capable of contributing to the improvement of health-services and the control of health-service costs are to be properly developed. For its part the Commission has indicated, on many different occasions – and in a variety of different ways, its willingness to play a part in making it possible for member-state health-care systems to work more closely together.

It is, however, a different story when it comes to member-states. Member states have been much less enthusiastic about the kinds of international collaborations and relationships that academics and health specialists have called for. In the case of the UK common European endeavours frequently attract a poor press. So far as health services are concerned member-states, not just the UK, have been hard to interest and reluctant to enter into relationships with the European Commission that might lead on to arrangements which make the relative performance of their health services more transparent. This has been a major source of frustration – as indicated in an earlier chapter – for European parliamentarians whose support for an increased Commission budget, to implement the long delayed health monitoring programme, was rebuffed by the Council (BMJ, 1996a: 1060). Even those health ministers, who claim to be enthusiastic about strengthening the European Commission's input into health-care policy-making, carefully qualify their support (Jowell, 1998: 4). Politicians responsible for health services are, perhaps understandably, concerned about being portrayed by political rivals as favouring health-service bureaucracy over clinical services. Such concern is rightly questioned and hard to justify rationally – but that does not lessen its political significance (Croxson, 1999: 12–39). Anything that can be described as support for international bureaucracy presents a particularly attractive political target, however persuasively 'experts' make the case for funding international collaborations, joint research or information exchange. Member states are clearly unwilling to fund anything that might approach a state of the art EU collaboration, capable of sharing and developing knowledge of health service effectiveness and ushering in an age of evidence based medicine from the Atlantic to the Urals.

The new EU Health Commissioner, David Byrne, claimed that he was 'realistic' about the prospects of getting additional resources to support EU health-policy activities. In a written reply, to a European Parliamentary Question, submitted in advance of the confirmation hearings for new Commissioners in 1999, Mr Byrne explained that:

> The Berlin European Council has determined the financial allocations for Community policies for the whole period of the new Commission ... I think it essential therefore that we make the best use we can of the resources at our disposal.
>
> (EU Confirm, 1999: 19)

Despite the parsimony, which often characterises national government decisions about funding international bodies, the case for better funded international collaborations, in which the European Commission could play an enhanced role, has been made with great conviction by academic health-policy specialists (Figueras and Saltman, 1998: 99–101). And dramatic advances are being made in developing the *information super-highway* capable of facilitating information exchange. An electronic highway which already makes it possible for complex and extended exchanges of information to take place between scientists, professionals, public officials and others who are based in different countries.

The potential impact of the *information highway* on public sector activities

International communication networks have the potential to dramatically lower the costs of working together – sharing information and exchanging views – over great distances. Technological advances are not only reducing the costs of computing and of telecommunications they are greatly extending the capabilities of data exchange systems. The European Commission itself claims to be convinced that the digital revolution in communications can reshape and improve governance, enhance the possibilities for exchanging information between governments, public-service providers and the general public and greatly expand opportunities for sharing new knowledge. Information technology is increasingly being presented as a key to building European society and making life better for all Europeans. Indeed the Commission has sought to evangelise on behalf of the new *information society*. It has become a proselytiser, urging Europeans to embrace the information age not only in commerce but also in the service of the public. Something that the Commission's Green Paper, entitled *Public Sector Information: A Key Resource for Europe*, makes plain (CEC, 1998e). It would surely be unwise to disagree with those who believe that the impact of contemporary and 21st century information technologies will ultimately be felt more strongly in the public services than in the fields of private communication, commerce or entertainment.

The aims of this chapter and of the Commission

In this Chapter the reader will be offered an account of the EC's efforts to encourage and foster the development of health telematics and to improve information systems for health, health-care providers, managers and medical researchers and patients in the EU. The chapter is also designed to provide the reader with an account of the attempts made by the European Commission to influence and steer the European health-policy agenda. The Commission, most notably the former Social Affairs Commissioner Padraig Flynn, has attempted to persuade member-states that there is a strong case for equipping the Commission – or quite possibly other international organisations, with which the Commission could work closely – with the ability to serve as a clearing house for health information and analysis. The Commission has sought, with limited success, to get member-states to give it the authority and to provide it with the resources needed to play a constructive role in assisting them to learn from one another, by sharing information about the health of their populations and the strengths and weaknesses, successes and failures, of their health services. The Commission has argued that there is a European imperative to make the most effective use of the public funds that are spent on health services. It accepts that expenditure on health services is substantial and exceptionally difficult to restrain. Health spending has grown rapidly in the past and may grow strongly again. Growth of health spending can profoundly affect tax levels and the economic competitiveness of member-states. The Commission has supported the view that if European societies fail to develop their capacity to make the best of their health-care resources they risk losing their ability to sustain equitable health-care systems and will almost certainly be unable to strengthen the European *social model*. The distinctiveness of EU societies is held, in part, to be a function of the European social model. A model that entails the removal or lowering of financial barriers to accessing health services. Indeed accessible and equitable health-care are considered to be at the core of the European social model.

   Interpreted in this way the role, in facilitating the efficient and effective management of health-care systems, which the Commission has been seeking, becomes part of an intensely political project. Its purpose – set against the background of an avalanche of health-care system reforms in OECD countries, including EU member-states – is to uphold longstanding commitments to equity and universality in European health-care systems.

A case of advancing when and where you can

The European Commission has been forbidden from taking a direct hand in the management of member-state health-care systems but encouraged by Treaty to assist member-states to work together to find ways, collaboratively and co-operatively, to improve their health-care systems. Programmes designed to encourage scientific collaborations have tended to be less controversial in member-states – and better funded – than programmes aimed explicitly at promoting social and economic collaboration between member-states in the health and welfare fields. The European Commission, on behalf of the EC, enjoyed considerable scope to promote and support scientific research and technological development in member-states. This has included support for medical research and the development of information technologies. A reflection, perhaps, of the approach established under EURATOM to activities perceived as highly technical and economically promising.

The EC/EU and the development of health-related information systems

Beginning with AIM, which stands for Advanced Informatics in Medicine, the EC/EU has invested considerable sums in the development of information systems for use in medicine and health-care. Community funded research and development work on health-information systems has been extraordinarily diverse and wide-ranging. Something that is reflected in the baffling array of acronyms used to describe EC/EU medical and health-information projects. AIM was initiated in the late 1980s, with large numbers of research projects and initiatives being established in the early 1990s. In part AIM can be represented as a response to mounting anxiety about the lack of European competitiveness in markets for new technologies. It was also justified as a European investment capable of seeding the process of innovation in member-states and securing continent wide improvements in medical care and health services. AIM formed part of the European Community's third Framework Programme for European research; it has, with successor programmes, been a contribution to European Research and Technological Development (R&TD) activities. In the words of the final report on AIM:

> It was ... realised that the largest public sector in the EC, i.e. the health-care sector with 8–10% of GNP, was introducing informatics and communication tools somewhat lacking in co-ordination, even at local and regional level. This left the sector fragmented, hard to access for European vendors, and difficult to use as a base for world market expansion. ... An exploratory AIM action ran from 1988 to 1990 to encourage co-ordination in the EC of health-care developments. ... Notable examples of relying on telematics were coming from the other side of the Atlantic. In the USA, in October 1992 it had been decided that major improvements in patient data communication and reimbursement schemes based on modern telematics would be implemented gradually from 1994. ... [AIM had an EC] budget of 97 million ECU. This was seen as probably the minimum financial volume to keep the interest of commercial actors in a user driven programme. According to the Council Decision the objective was *"to*

stimulate the development of harmonised applications of information and communication technologies in health-care and to develop a European health-care information infrastructure taking into account the needs of users and technological opportunities".

(Sosa-Iudicissa, 1996: vol. 1, 3; emphasis added)

In 1992 AIM consisted of '37 cost-shared projects ... about 300 partners, 5 concerted actions with more than 100 participants, and ... links to industry, telecom services, health-care providers, research institutions, and the Comité Européean de Normalisation (CEN), the European standardisation organisation' (ibid., 3). AIM was succeeded by the EU *health telematics programme* and funded as part of the fourth European Framework Programme for R&TD. The latest iteration of EU R&TD activities, the fifth Framework Programme, will include a major health-related research component, designed to build on earlier support for the development of medical and health-care information systems.

A major investment in health-information systems

Majorie Gott's (1995) *Telematics for Health – the Role of telehealth and Telemedicine in Homes and Communities*, reflects the impact and importance, in terms of Community funded research, of the development work commissioned by the EC/EU in supporting the application of new technologies, particularly electronic technologies, to health. As she points out: 'Telematics in Health Care was by far the largest [EC] programme ... [it included work on] diagnosis and surveillance for clinical decision making ... fetal monitoring and diabetic self-care' (21). EC/EU research funds – expended under the third and fourth research frameworks – have supported numerous IT projects, programmes and activities relevant to health-care services and systems. DGXIII, responsible for the European Commission's applied research programme, has proudly displayed, on one of its web pages, details of European Marrow Donor Information System (EMDIS) under the title '*101 Telematics Applications Success Stories*'. EMDIS is proclaimed as an EU health telematics success:

More than half of the hundreds of patients needing bone marrow transplants have not been able to find donors in their own country. No single country has the resources to build up a national donor registry of sufficient size for all its patients. EMDIS was established to address this problem. Working in a dozen of countries, EMDIS has facilitated and streamlined international co-operation and communication between

Box 7.1 A sample of the dozens of EC/EU-funded health telematics projects

RACE (Research and Development in Advance Communications Technologies in Europe) was intended to develop telephony services for people with special needs.

TIDE (Technology Initiative for Disabled and Elderly people) was an initiative aimed at supporting and developing the European market for rehabilitation technologies.

HELIOS (Handicapped People in the European Community Living in an Open Society) was intended to make new technologies serve people with disabilities and enable them to live as fully as possible as members of society.

AORTICS (Advanced Open Resources Telematics in Critical Care Situations) was intended to support the use of advanced information systems in providing critical care.

COCO (Co-ordination and Continuity in Primary Care – the regional healthcare information network) was aimed at improving co-ordination in primary care services.

EUROPATH (European Pathology Assisted by Telematics) was designed to assist the development of pathology services in Europe.

national registries of volunteer bone marrow donors. The project has provided the impetus for defining EU standards and encouraged co-operation and creation of a European system for identifying suitable donors.

The full titles of programmes, typically known by their acronyms, gives some idea of the range of health information systems development work which the EC/EU has supported.

Substantial investment of variable quality

The overall quality and utility of such diverse research and development programmes for health-information systems is hard to assess. Those responsible for commissioning new research and development projects, for the EU's fifth Framework Programme, have sought to increase the rigour of the processes for considering proposals and assessing results and have emphasised the importance attached to the practical benefits projects are expected to produce. It is evident, in the documents describing the goals of EU research for the 21st century, that EU funded work on information systems for health-care is expected to demonstrate direct relevance to the delivery of health services. The Commission's DGXII claims that the fifth Framework Programme for research (FP5) '... differs considerably from its predecessors. It has been conceived to help solve problems and to respond to the major socio-economic challenges facing Europe'. The Commission's 1999 Annual Report on the Research and Technological Development activities of the EU claimed that: 'The new [FP] concentrates resources ... on 23 key actions *meeting the priority needs of society*, paying particular attention to the potential for applying the results'. (CEC, 1999b: 2).

IT and pressures for the convergence and reformation of health-care systems

Is work on health telematics part of a much heralded convergence of interests and of technologies destined to make it increasingly attractive (and urgent) for providers and planners of health services to support and employ increasingly powerful information systems? As the size of professional, managerial, research and client communities that share information increases, differences in performance will quickly become noticeable. The same arrangements which ensure that others have better access to information about what you are doing will also provide you with much better information about what they are doing. In circumstances where the pressure to make better use of health-care resources has been increasing, information systems themselves make comparisons easier and more potent. It does not seem unreasonable to expect that improvements in information systems might accelerate the rate at which improvements in practice and resource management spread.

According to this – some would say – optimistic view of the positive and self-reinforcing role of contemporary information systems, the EC can claim to have provided some of the early leadership and to have supported pioneering work in the field of health telematics.

Telematics – a neologism constructed from two words, *tele*communications and infor*matics* – refers to '... the sudden expansion of telecommunications technologies which allow computers ... to communicate with each other ... in such a way as to enable virtually instant access to remote neworks' (de Dombal, 1996: 24). Tim de Dombal was, until his death in 1995, a leading figure in the development of medical information systems. He was in no doubt that a revolution in health-care was underway and that the 'impact [of telematics] on medicine ... [would] be considerable'. It is likely that even de Dombal would be surprised at what has now been made possible by utilising developments in digital and telecommunications technologies. He would undoubtedly be impressed by the burgeoning numbers of telematics applications to be found in medicine and health services management. Amongst those applications is telemedicine (Viegas and Dunn, 1998; Wootton and Craig, 1999). Telemedicine, 'medicine at a distance' (Wootton and Craig, 1999: 4), has been described as a development with remarkable potential to:

> address the key issues that challenge medical practice at the turn of the century: maximizing efficiency while maintaining or improving the quality of service, lowering costs, improving access to care, improving access to information, and assuring patient confidentiality and professional accountability. There is no other technique or systems engineering strategy that has the promise of addressing these issues in as global and cost-effective way as telemedicine.
>
> (Wootton and Craig, 1999: 3)

Telemedicine raises the possibility of medical services and health-care organised and delivered in ways that transcend national boundaries and existing health-care systems. It is, potentially, a mighty challenge to nation-state management and control of health-care systems and it is a subject we will return at the end of this chapter.

The Commission and information about health care and health-care systems

The idea that the European Commission has an important role to play in influencing and facilitating the development of health-policy in the EU has been vigorously promoted since the early 1990s. Three publications have been chosen to reflect different facets of the Commission's attempts to shape and contribute to a European health-policy agenda. All three publications, one of which resulted from a European Health Policy Conference, have helped to structure the discussion of issues in European health-care policy which follows (Abel-Smith *et al.*, 1995a; Jakubowski *et al.*, 1998; EHF, 1999).

Jakubowski and Busse on comparing EU health-care systems

The EU's Directorate General for Research – DGIII – commissioned Elke Jakubowski, an advisor based in the Public Health Policy Department of

Epidemiology and Social Medicine at the Medical School, Hannover – to write a report on the health-care systems of all 15 EU member-states. Jakubowski's report, intended to inform the work of the European Parliament, was published in November 1998 (SACO 101 EN). The report, entitled *Health Care Systems in the EU: a Comparative Study*, can itself be viewed as an attempt by the Commission to underpin and explain EU claims to a leading role in health information. A substantial amount of work is needed, in the words of the report, to focus co-operation between member-states on 'reshaping health-care systems', to direct them 'towards measurable outcomes such as quality of health-care' and to achieve higher levels of 'satisfaction amongst the population served' (Jakubowski *et al.*, 1998: 27).

Jakubowski begins her survey of the condition of European health-care systems by drawing attention to the Maastricht Treaty, which 'gave the EU new competences in public health and more scope for international co-operation' (Jakubowski *et al.*, 1998: 5). Jakubowski's introduction notes the Commission's role in health promotion and health protection and draws specific attention to an EU competence in 'subsidising ... medical and health-policy research, *and the establishment of international information systems'*. The case for the Commission to act as a partner for member-state health-policy development has – she claims – been given a further boost by the Treaty of Amsterdam. Taken together with the SEM, the Treaty encourages 'policy convergence' and the construction of 'new routes for the exchange of medical technology, health services and manpower resources' (Jakubowski *et al.*, 1998: 5). Jakubowski and her co-author, Reinhard Busse, make it plain that they believe that their report provides an account of European health systems at a watershed. 'Health care in the EU is [said to be] at a cross-roads', challenges and opportunities abound. This somewhat apocalyptic view was no doubt intended to dramatise policy choices and to focus attention on the condition of European health-care systems. Jakubowski and Busse set out to provide Members of the EP – (and others – their report is freely downloadable from the world wide web) – with a guide to the principal issues which they believe should concern Members of the EP and health-care policy-makers in all the member-states.

Time to act

Member states need, according to Jakubowski and Busse, to make the most of the opportunities that arise from the convergence of health-care systems. Highly centralised health-care systems, like the NHS in Britain, are said to be accepting and promoting the devolution of responsibility for service delivery as well as encouraging greater diversity of supply. Other states, where funding arrangements have traditionally been more varied and complex and which have always supported a diversity of providers, are seeking to manage overall spending on health services more strongly and improve co-ordination of services. Local autonomy is being encouraged on the one hand and greater central control of spending on the other. In other words health systems across Europe are seeking a more appropriate mix between national standard setting and local commissioning. In order to get the best from changes and developments, in the organisation and management of health-care systems, they suggest it is imperative that member-states appreciate that they are facing 'common challenges in delivering equal, efficient and high quality health services at affordable cost'. Being at the 'cross-roads' means there will be plenty of opportunities to share experiences and benefit from doing so (Jakubowski *et al.*, 1998: 5). Propositions and statements in support of increased Union collaboration litter their report (see Box 7.2).

Jakubowski *et al.'s* report is only the latest in a series of reports and speeches that have sought to press the case for a EU-wide health-policy and information resource and to frame a European health-policy agenda. Most promote the idea of an honest broker – able to work with health-care systems across the Union – and are committed to the maintenance of the European social model in health.

Flynn promotes the Commission

Padraig Flynn has been particularly assiduous in making the case for European health-policy collaboration and encouraging others to do so. He wrote the foreword to *Choices in Health Policy: an Agenda for the European Union* (Abel-Smith *et al.*, 1995). In many ways it is a seminal publication, intended to mark out common ground for would be EU health-policy collaborators. *Choices in Health Policy*, published jointly by the Office for Official Publications of the European Communities and Dartmouth Publishing Company, is described in its opening pages as a contribution to European Political Economy. A somewhat provocative designation for a publication based squarely on a research study commissioned by European Commission.

The themes found in Flynn's foreword, to *Choices in Health Policy*, have been maintained throughout his time in office as the EU Commissioner for Social Affairs. His enthusiasm for European collaboration, apparent in the foreword to *Choices in Health Policy*, was also evident in his contribution to the inaugural conference of the European Health Forum – Gastein, held in Austria in 1998. The Forum appears to have been

Box 7.2   Selective quotations from Elke Jakubowski and Reinhard Busse's EU Parliamentary Working Paper Comparing EU member state health-care systems – setting a European health policy agenda?

1. '. . . information on health and health care can be circulated more rapidly.' (1998: 6).
2. 'Each system has its own strengths and weaknesses and none of the systems provides a wholly successful solution. Hence each has something to learn from the experience of the other fourteen [EU Member State health care systems]' (1998: 6).
3. 'The standardisation of data definitions and methods of data collection has not yet been fully realised, though subject to substantial international effort' (1998: 6).
4. 'The quantification and qualification of health is a prerequisite for the identification of population health need and the translation into health care provision' (1998: 9).
5. '. . . advances in medical science will give rise to new demand for health care by increasing the capacity to prevent, diagnose, treat, cure and rehabilitate disease . . . [While] [t]echnolog[ical] innovation for health care promotes the industrial sector and has tremendous potential to reduce costs . . . health care technology resources are not always deployed in an optimal fashion: wasteful provision and utilisation by those who provide and utilise health care technology is often attributed to a lack of cost-consciousness' (1998: 10 & 21).
6. '. . . cross-country comparisons of health status indices are only valid within the limits of data availability and comparability' (1998: 10).
7. 'The aim is to share the costs of medical care between the sick and the well and to adjust for different levels of ability to pay. This mechanism of solidarity reflects consensus in the European Union that health care should not be left to a free market alone.' (1998:10).
8. 'Variations in health care expenditure and resources among EU Member States suggest that there are many different ways of achieving the same objective and thus a broad scope for comparison of international experience of getting the best value for money' (1998: 11).
9. 'Internationally comparable morbidity data are scarce and often lack reliability' (1998: 16).

Box 7.2   *continued*

10. 'There is a lack of availability of reliable and recent comparable data on health care input factors and utilisation rates. Provision and utilisation of hospital care differs by up to a factor of six in the European Union Member States but country data are highly controversial among different sources' (1998: 22).

11. 'In terms of health care productivity, hospital data are in favour of those countries with a comparatively low number of inpatient beds, namely the UK and Denmark . . . the level of doctors, nurses, pharmacists and dentists . . . show a striking diversity in the countries of the EU' (1998: 23 & 24).

12. 'Greater cost effectiveness is seen as a route for more health care per Euro. . . . The search for increased efficiency implies the search for improved or stable quality service provision within given financial limits. . . . This might require . . . health care systems to integrate [information about] population [health] into the process of establishing standards for quality care. This also requires good quality comparable information on patients treated, on outcome and costs of health care and from the reform of the system' (1998: 26).

Source: European Parliament – Directorate General for Research, Working Paper – Health Care in the EU a Comparative Study – Public Health and Consumer Protection Series SACO 101 EN – November-1998.

conceived, with Flynn's strong support, as a vehicle for debate about EU health policies and its health competence. Padraig Flynn told the conference that:

> The EU has a role in helping governments address [the challenges confronting contemporary health-care systems] by providing good, comparable information and high quality analysis, by establishing best practice and disseminating it, and by developing supportive European legislation.
>
> (EHF, 1998: 151)

The basic argument was presented in Flynn's foreword to *Choices in Health Policy* and repeated at Gastein, in 1998. European nations face severe problems in managing their medical care systems and responding to the health needs of their citizens. Member states could benefit substantially by enabling the Commission to co-ordinate the exchange of information between them and to contribute to the analysis of health-policy. Concerted action and co-operation between member states is essential if health-care reforms are to be carried through successfully – without imperilling the principles upon which European health-care systems have hitherto rested.

The arguments were intended to have a wide appeal. Member-state governments were certainly in Flynn's sights but so were Europe's citizens and health-care professionals and managers. In 1995 Flynn had claimed that the 'Health policy and health systems in the European Union [were] at a critical juncture'. There were 'enormous challenges to be overcome'. He identified them as responding to:

- demographic change;
- increasing population mobility;
- growing problems of social exclusion;
- mounting problems in meeting the cost of expensive new therapeutic techniques;
- increasing pressures (and difficulties in responding to pressures) to satisfy rising public demands and expectations of health-care systems.

Europeans needed to understand that these challenges were not insurmountable. In fact there were 'new opportunities to meet and overcome those challenges and secure substantial improvements in health'. Among the new opportunities was the '. . . coming into effect of the Treaty on European Union . . . [it provided for] . . . international co-operation and for Union-wide initiatives *which [could] provide all Member States with access to the very best expertise and the greatest experience available'* (Abel-Smith *et al.*, 1995, xi).

The fact that he was making essentially the same appeal and presenting essentially the same arguments some four years later can be interpreted in a variety of ways. Is it evidence of the strength of a convinced European's belief in the importance and continued efficacy of the European social model? Certainly it is. Is it evidence of his limited success in influencing member states to support more ambitious health policies? Certainly it is that as well.

The former European Commissioner, responsible for Employment and Social Affairs, took the opportunity afforded by introducing *Choices in Health Policy* to applaud the Ministers of Health, who had, at a special meeting in Rhodes in May of 1994, considered the report produced for the

Commission by Abel-Smith and his team. The report urged member states to work together in order to address 'fundamental health choices'. The report was presented as evidence that the Commission could take the lead. The fact that Ministers of Health had met together to discuss it was presented, rather less convincingly, as a sign that member states were prepared to be persuaded of the necessity to support an enhanced role for the Commission. Commissioner Flynn described the report itself as an 'authoritative survey of the main determinants of health status in the Union . . . the organisation of health services and the issues that member states have to address in framing their policies for the future'. But perhaps the key purpose of the report was to establish a convincing European health-policy agenda that had the unequivocal support of health-policy experts and specialists. *Choices in Health Policy*, he wrote, identified: 'the areas where the European Community can play a valuable and complementary role [to health-policy making in Member States] . . .'. What were the areas Flynn's experts had identified?

Information and health – the issues facing member states

In their introduction to the report Abel-Smith and his colleagues asserted that their recommendations focused on 'two main issues facing Member States':

1. How to obtain further health improvements.
2. How to secure greater efficiency in the use of health resources.

They observed that: [While the] 'organisation and financing of health-care differs considerably between Member States', as does the provision of resources 'such as doctors and hospital beds' and the utilisation of services, they had not been able to discover any consistent relationship between what was known about variations in provision and use of services *and* death rates (Abel-Smith *et al.*, 1995: xix). In short, the authors of this seminal report, on fundamental choices in European health-policy-making, claimed that despite the very substantial and rising cost of medical-care services and health-care systems next to nothing was known about the relationships between health-system inputs and outputs. In the context of diverse and increasingly expensive health-care systems, supported by large sums of public money, the case for investing in health research and information systems, which would help policy-makers to explore the differences between health-care systems, in order to inform decisions about them, seemed irresistible.

Health system reforms galore

The publication of *Choices in Health Policy*, in 1995, came hard on the heels of what Mia Defever described as the emergence of international trends in health-policy reform apparent throughout Western societies (1995: 1–7). By 1995 major health-care reforms were underway or contemplated in almost all OECD (Organisation for Economic co-operation and Development) countries. Reform programmes appeared similar, although the reform process itself could also be characterised as somewhat contradictory. It included support for local or devolved management of health-services and a great tightening up of national controls on health-service expenditures. Quasi-market developments were combined with a relaxation of some central controls – but budgets for providing services were, while being managed locally, subject to firm centrally determined disciplines and limits. Defever's view was that 'concern about the reduction of public deficits [was] prevailing over attention to cost-effectiveness of the [health-care systems] . . .' (1995: 5). Defever's review of health-care reforms was subtitled *the unfinished agenda*. The predominance of political and financial considerations in shaping the reform process was interpreted as evidence that:

> The State is not a neutral arbiter among competing groups, but a self-interested actor itself, making alliances with other major interest groups, resulting in policies which are not necessarily in the public interest.
>
> (Defever, 1995: 3).

An agenda for Europe

Abel-Smith and his associates, many of whom continue to research European health-care systems and to offer advice to European governments, subtitled their report *An Agenda for the European Union*. Their professional purpose seemed clear, to convince all those prepared to listen that it was necessary to inform the health-policy-making process by identifying and exploring fundamental questions about health and health services, before taking any major decisions about the organisation of health-care systems. Although their report, in its published form, had been labelled a work of political economy it concentrated on making the case for a more scientific, rational and empirical approach to health-policy making. It took the improvement of the European social model in health-care as its starting point; accepting, as the OECD had done, that maintaining access to health services, irrespective of the ability to pay, was a basic tenet of health service organisation in the advanced democracies (OECD, 1994).

Scepticism about the politics of health reform

There can be little doubt that the majority of health-policy academics and specialists are deeply sceptical about the politics of health service reform. They share Defever's view that 'policy choices are often not made on rational grounds with an optimal outcome' (1995: 3). Alan Maynard and Karen Bloor suggest, to borrow a phrase from Rudolf Klein, that elected politicians who have contributed to the 'global epidemic' of health-care reform, are generally unreceptive to informed argument about health reform. They characterise politicians' contributions to the health-policy debate as confused and muddled and unlikely to 'inform difficult choices' (Maynard and Bloor, 1995: 247–64, 1995). One of the principal propositions, advanced by the authors of *Choices in Health Policy*, is that we are all – public, politicians and health-policy-makers – ill-equipped to make choices in health-policy. And we are likely to remain so unless decisions are taken to improve sources of information about health and health-care and the ability to make use of the information collected. Perhaps this helps to explain why references to fundamental choices – in *Choices in Health Policy* – can appear confusing.

Critical and important choices (rather than fundamental choices)

The phrase fundamental choices may conjure up an image of decisions being made about whether or not to fund health-care systems out of general taxation. Most health-policy academics and health economists find proposals for the wholesale replacement of public revenues with private payments and medical insurance wholly unconvincing. The *fundamental choices* which occupy the minds of health-policy academics and researchers do not turn out – in the vast majority of cases – to be all that fundamental. Most of the contributors to the European Health Forum conference held in 1998, for example, focused their attention on trying to illuminate ways of managing public resources and health policies more successfully. It seemed they were convinced that the primary responsibility for funding and managing health-care should lie in the public domain. References, at the European Health Forum – Gastein, to major changes in the funding arrangement for health-care systems were largely confined to pointing out that expansion of private medical provision and payment systems were most unlikely to relieve the state of the need to raise substantial revenues. Indeed there were shared anxieties that such developments would inflate medical costs generally rather than contain them (EHF, 1999).

Questions facing health-policy-makers

The common and critical concerns, which the authors of *Choices in Health Policy* link with health-care choices, can best be represented by questions about the things that seem certain to continue to affect the delivery, organisation and effectiveness of health services most strongly. Questions to which, in most cases, we have only very sketchy and unsatisfactory answers. The questions can be formulated and spun in a variety of different ways:

1. Can we do better *and* keep the lid on health-care spending? What are the best ways of containing health-care costs?
2. Are there health-system reforms that can preserve what we value about our health services and still equip them to do a better job? How are health-system reforms, cost-containment and an emphasis on cost-effectiveness related to one another? How far can they be reconciled with one another?
3. What are the best ways to improve the effectiveness of health services? Can we develop the means to speed up the dissemination and adoption of the most cost-effective ways of providing services?
4. Is it possible to differentiate between 'new medical advances', so that we become better at picking and backing therapeutic winners and resisting medical innovations of little worth? How should scientific and technological developments relevant to the delivery of health services be assessed?
5. How should health-service priorities be set? Are there better ways of making difficult choices about allocating scarce resources? Is it possible to develop greater public understanding of the need to plan services and determine priorities?
6. Is it possible to achieve a better balance between different kinds of health services? How should the balance between different kinds of health-care interventions (for example – curative, preventive, and educational health services) be determined?
7. Are there better ways of planning and delivering services to people who need them but have little or no political clout? What choices are there

in designing, developing and implementing health services to meet the health-care needs of particular groups such as migrants, the poor, the mentally ill and the elderly?

Proposals – for Europe's health agenda

In the ninth and final chapter of the published version of their report to the Commission Abel-Smith and his collaborators set out their 'Proposals for the Future Role of the European Community' (1995, 125–43). They made 23 proposals or recommendations. They were in no doubt, having reviewed the legislative framework under which the Commission was expected to operate post-Maastricht and considered the kinds of issues and questions that policy-makers needed to address, that there was:

- a demonstrable need for health-policy co-ordination, which the Commission was well placed to provide;

they believed that they had identified:

- clear opportunities, which the Commission was best placed to exploit, for member states to learn from each others experiences;

and,

- reason to believe that the Commission could act more cheaply, on behalf of the Community, than member states could acting on their own.

They had found:

- persuasive evidence that issues that cross national boundaries can be more appropriately dealt with by the Commission than by member states acting in isolation;
- a good case for developing and employing standard definitions, where member states need to or are required to share and exchange information;
- evidence that action and policies have implications for health and well-being that go beyond the boundaries of individual member states.

The nub of the case for a more active Commission was to be found in the fact that, as the report put it, 'the majority of health-care interventions are unevaluated or inadequately evaluated . . . [and there is a limited supply], within Europe, of individuals with the skills required to undertake high quality health service research' (Abel-Smith *et al.*, 1995: 129–30). Health outcomes research and health technology assessment work, of high quality, would only be possible if there was a determined effort to concentrate it 'in carefully chosen centres so as to achieve economies of scale and develop training centres'. European initiatives, from which all the member states might benefit and to which they could contribute appropriately, would maximise the benefits derived for all parties and 'avoid duplication of effort' (Abel-Smith *et al.*, 1995, 130). High quality information, capable of securing health improvements and more cost-effective use of health service resources, would increase the incentive to put in place the systems needed for exchanging information between health systems and health-policy makers.

Some problems with making comparisons to inform policy

However, making health-systems comparisons is not at all straight-forward. The extent of confusion about the meaning and significance of international health comparisons is easy to illustrate. The case for improving the quality of information, in order to counter crude and misleading presentations of comparative health data is also easy to illustrate. And, given the scepticism among academic health-policy specialists about the political process and nervousness about the susceptibilities of politicians responsible for major health-policy decisions, it is also easy to understand why many social scientists and epidemiologists are strongly committed to investing heavily in improving health data and raising the general level of debate about health-policy issues.

A British tabloid reports on basic health-systems data

A British tabloid newspaper report, in August 1999, serves as a good example of the poor quality of existing comparative health data and the insupportable burden that it is often made to carry. When the *Daily Mail*, said to be the most important tabloid read for Britain's Prime Minister, Tony Blair, headlined news of health data published by the Office of Health Economics (OHE), in the OHE's Compendium of Health Statistics for 1999, it underscored the political sensitivity of statistics about health services. The *Daily Mail's* headline declared that OHE data showed 'Britain Bottom of the Health League' (*Daily Mail*, Friday, 13 August 1999).

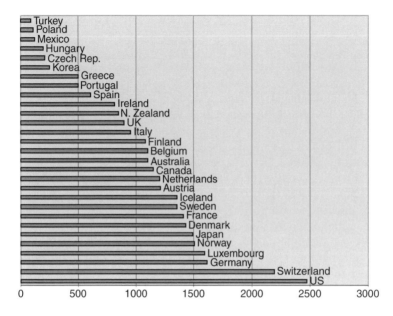

Figure 7.1 Total health spend per person in 1997, by country (*Daily Mail* chart excluded countries with a lower spend per head than the UK)
Sources: Based on: *Daily Mail*, 13 August 1999, OHE Compendium, 11th Edition, 1999 and OECD health data.

Being bottom of any league, let alone a health league, cannot be an enjoyable experience for a national political leader. The *Daily Mail's* evidence for its claim – that the UK was in last place – was somewhat less convincing than the opinions of sports journalists about the position of football teams in football league tables. Football league tables do have an unambiguous relationship to wins and losses and goals scored and conceded. In the *Daily Mail's* health league tables the relationship between performance and position was represented as equally self-evident. But, does low health-service spending equal poor performance? While the UK was ranked bottom of just 18 selected countries, in a table arranged according to annual expenditure on health per head of population, it is far from certain that good health is closely related to high levels of spending on health-care. The UK was also shown near the foot of a hospital beds league table. In a table, made up of 24 countries, the UK was shown to have fewer hospital inpatient beds per 1,000 population than the Czech Republic, Greece or Korea; the UK was just third from bottom. The *Daily Mail's* inside page report, entitled 'Sick at heart, our

NHS', included a third table, showing coronary heart disease death rates for men and women aged between 45 and 64. In this case – as with golf scores – lower death rates were interpreted as evidence of good performance. While the *Daily Mail* story focussed on the UK, with the ninth highest coronary mortality rates, it neglected the data presented for the USA. And America, shown at the top of the expenditure league table, was at the bottom of the hospital beds table. A somewhat puzzling result, if good performance is to be equated with having more hospital beds. In the third of the *Daily Mail's* health league tables, for coronary heart disease, the USA was shown to be performing better than the UK. Even so the US was shown to have the eleventh highest coronary death rate out of 27 nations. Putting all three tables together the reader could be forgiven for wondering whether, with spending three times more per head per annum, the American's league positions helped or hindered the case for increasing expenditure on health-care in Britain. The careful reader would, for instance, have noted that Korea had done best. With a similar provision of hospital beds per 1,000 population to the UK it had the lowest coronary mortality rates for men and women of any of the countries represented in the tables. Korea did not appear at all in the table showing health expenditure per head of population. While the *Daily Mail* can be criticised for selective presentation of international health data and for drawing conclusions, from the data, that were wholly unjustified the information displayed on its pages is representative of the international data sets constructed by the OECD from information supplied by national governments. Unless the quality and comparability of the health information governments collect and exchange is dramatically improved it will continue to be of little use to national health-policy-makers who hope to do better by learning from others about what they do better.

The fundamental proposition contained in *Choices for Health Policy*, placed before health ministers from EU member states at Rhodes in 1994, was quite simply that without good information on health care effectiveness, 'to inform purchasing and planning decisions', it will not be possible improve the use made of the scarce public resources employed in providing health services.

Others enter the ring

The factors, which have made it difficult, for the European Commission, to implement key recommendations contained in *Choices in Health Policy*, may help to explain developments at WHO – European Regional Office. WHO (European Region) has closely allied itself with a new European

Health Observatory designed to improve international health data and research. The OECD has been emphasising its interest in playing an enhanced role in the measurement of health outcomes. And other EU institutions, most notably and perhaps rather surprisingly the European Investment Bank (EIB), have demonstrated a willingness to promote and support work which the Commission might, if it had been better supported and more appropriately resourced, have undertaken in-house.

The difficulties that the Commission has had in making progress with the proposal, contained in its principal Communication on health policy in the early 1990s (CEC, 1993b), to build a health-monitoring system, provide an insight into the obstacles the Commission has faced (and continues to encounter) in establishing itself as an effective partner for member-state health-care statistical services and information systems.

In her report, *European Union Health Policy on the Eve of the Millennium*, Lyndsay Mountford provides an account of an EU project that appears to have become a growing source of frustration and embarrassment for almost all of those involved. In many organisational surveys and reports it is necessary to read between the lines – in this case little is left to the reader's imagination:

2.52 Health monitoring (is) ... widely seen as an important and prospectively valuable tool, but its implementation appears to have been a particular source of difficulty to international collaborators and member states alike ... 2.53 A logical progression in the development of a system of data collection would have been (a) identification of data set, (b) definition of terms and collection standards, (c) transfer arrangements. Instead, the EU has already established the Interchange of Data between Administrations (IDA) project, which divides into the HSSCD (Health Surveillance System for Communicable Diseases) electronic network for the exchange of information on communicable diseases, and HIEMS (Health Indicators Exchange and Monitoring System). It is extremely difficult to know how electronic data could be developed or justified, ahead of having identified the relevant data set and, depending on how extensive this is, the most cost-effective means of transferring it. Several commentators queried the value for money of HIEMS.

(Mountford, 1998a: 19–20).

The launch of the European Observatory on Health Care in February 1999, with the WHO as its first named partner and sponsor, and with firm backing from the EIB, has been described as an attempt to 'bridge the gap between academia and policy makers' (Richards, 1999). It can also be interpreted as a consequence of mounting frustration with other attempts to develop collaborative work on health monitoring and health-information systems. One of the Observatory's directors and the co-ordinator of its activities, Josep Figueras, has argued consistently that health-care reforms in Europe have been influenced more strongly by ideology than by analyses of the results of policy changes and organisational reform (Figueras and Saltman, 1998).

The importance attached to work of the kind Joseph Figueras now co-ordinates can be gauged from the ringing endorsement for undertaking it supplied by Sir Brian Unwin, President of the EIB. In an article published in *Eurohealth* in August 1999 Sir Brian, who begins by proclaiming the EIB's financial strength, goes on to add that the EIB now has responsibilities and a mandate to undertake projects which 'are not only financially sound but also socially worthwhile' (Unwin, 1999). Since 1997 the EIB has been authorised to support investment in both healthcare and education. The EIB's support for the European Observatory is described by Sir Brian as part of the Bank's strategy to 'establish a series of ... partnerships with individuals and organisations at the "leading edge"'. The Bank has identified the Observatory as a partner able to play a leading role in informing its health-care investment decisions and assisting it to develop and apply a 'health gain test' (Unwin, 1999: 8). The challenge, to health-policy makers and the EIB itself, is, according to Sir Brian, 'to find ways of using EIB resources for innovative projects that promote better integration across the primary, secondary and tertiary levels of health care'.

The European Observatory on Health Care Systems was not set up as an EU agency, reporting directly to the Commission, but its other partners, the Government of Norway, the Government of Spain, two Schools of the University of London and The World Bank, suggest that it is well placed to offer a lead to those in member states and the Commission who want health-policy reform to rest upon more secure empirical foundations.

Melissa Jee and Zeynep Or, responsible for an influential OECD occasional paper on health indicators, reinforce the case for 'better information on health outcomes' and champion an approach which focuses attention on outcomes and outcome-oriented policy making (OECD,1999). They lament the 'lack of international consensus on the concepts of health and morbidity ... [on] methodology and administration ... [which make] international comparisons next to impossible' (OECD,1999: para. 9). The standardisation of health measures to facilitate the exchange of information and comparisons between different countries could, they suggest, be undertaken by the OECD (para. 24). Given the importance of such work, to improving understanding of health outcomes, they suggest it is largely a question of whether OECD member states are prepared to provide sufficient resources to enable the OECD Secretariat to (para 27):

- build an international collaboration and establish a common set of health measures relevant to assessing the 'performance of medical-care systems';
- obtain the agreements needed to standardise concepts and definitions of health;
- obtain the agreements needed to standardise concepts and definitions of health-system performance;
- encourage and support application of agreed concepts and definitions;
- encourage and support analytical work utilising the common data set created;
- collaborate with other international organisations and initiatives (WHO and Eurostat – the statistical arm of the EU Commission are specifically mentioned).

In concluding their OECD occasional paper Jee and Orr summarise initiatives and projects which the OECD could launch subject, once again, to 'sufficient resources being made available' (para. 172):

- organise a network of experts in interested countries to help with the work;
- undertake a critical review of the current state of knowledge;
- propose a framework for developing international indicators for a limited set of conditions.

A continuing reluctance to invest and an expert view of the issues

National governments remain reluctant to invest the sums needed to construct worthwhile international health databases oriented towards the comparative assessment of health-service effectiveness. They have been much more enthusiastic about applying what might be called health-reform nostrums to the management of health-care budgets. Such nostrums – which include controls on payments for common procedures, introducing user charges or making greater use of them, controlling the supply of key health personnel, introducing cash-limited budgets and exposing providers to competition – can all be made to look rather like quack remedies for dealing with the alleged problem of *swollen health budgets*.

Seasoned observers of the European health-care scene, such as Jef van Langendonck, have been critical of fashions in health-care policy-making which focus on general budgetary anxieties. His keynote contribution, to the European Health Forum – Gastein, was clearly designed to explain why health-system reform proposals, which concentrate our attention on redrawing boundaries between the public and the private sector or shifting the balance between publicly and privately funded health-care, are likely to prove unproductive. van Langendonck's review of measures to keep costs down leads him to the conclusion that:

> measures to limit expenditure on health care have failed. . . . Maybe the overall expenditure would have been slightly higher without these measures, but we do not believe that the difference would be very important . . . .
>
> (EHF, 1999: 60)

van Langendonck argues that the peculiarities of the health-care sector, which include inelasticity of demand, asymmetry of information between doctor and patient, the considerable problems encountered when assessing the quality and effectiveness of health services and strong public support for equity in health services, makes health care exceptionally difficult to manage and organise. He eschews so-called fundamental reforms and proposes measures targeted at regulating and improving the quality of care. Quality controls – which take account of the peculiarities of the health-care sector – offer the best chance of producing the best results for the public. Attempts at regulating demand will fail to restrain expenditure and they will result in less equitable heath services and increased social inequality. In his words: ' . . . every penny spent on bad quality care is a penny . . . too much', such expenditure 'should be eliminated' (EHF, 1999: 61). Resources that are being used inappropriately can be redirected. The pursuit of better quality care depends, according to van Langendonck, on devising an effective quality control system. Such a system would include arrangements for:

- collecting data in a reliable and comparable way;
- ensuring that well motivated professionals are involved in the supervision of services and are ready and able to apply strong sanctions against those whose work is judged to be unsatisfactory;

- ensuring that patients are as well informed as possible about the choices that are open to them;
- a no-fault medical insurance scheme which would help to ensure that medical records could be used as quickly and constructively as possible to improve the quality of care generally.

Jef van Langendonck's message is quite clear. Political leaders and others who have the unenviable responsibility for determining the budgetary ceilings for health-care programmes should not confuse – nor should they be allowed to confuse – the management of overall spending on health care with the regulation of health care. It may be politically expedient to muddle the issues but – in van Langendonck's view – it simply serves to distract attention from the challenge of establishing the most effective quality control system possible. Jef van Langendonck was in no doubt about the benefits of: ' ... a co-ordinated European approach, instead of separate and mutually incompatible measures taken by individual countries' (EHF, 1999: 63).

A rival view – European health-care systems under threat

The health-policy agenda proposed and promoted at Gastein – Salzburg Austria, by the majority of contributors to the European Health Forum, has not gone unchallenged. In particular many find the idea that European governments can cope with all the changes affecting European health care systems on their own, even if they approach them more intelligently, unconvincing. In late July 1999 the *Healthcare Parliamentary Monitor* carried a story entitled 'Private healthcare in the EU faces "explosive growth"' (*HPM*, 1999: 15). The *Monitor* offered an account of an Economist Intelligence Unit (EIU) report on *The Prospects of Private Healthcare in Europe*. The EIU document, clearly aimed at an exclusive commercial audience, was priced at £775.00 per copy. It was said to have concluded that: '... throughout Western Europe it is becoming increasingly clear that public healthcare systems are no longer sustainable'.

The *Monitor* referred to research, 'conducted in six major European countries', which the EIU believed supported the view that 'Government-backed healthcare in Western Europe [was] in turmoil'. Publicly financed health-care systems were under assault. They were being undermined by: 'insatiable consumer demand', 'bloated hospital infrastructures', 'escalating medical costs', the 'swelling ranks of elderly people', the imposition of fiscal disciplines – to meet the Maastricht convergence criteria – and the development of new 'telecommunications technologies'. The new telecommunications technologies would make things even more difficult for existing publicly financed and managed health-care systems. Because they were bound to make health-care systems more transparent they would make it even harder to satisfy rising public expectations. The logic of the EIU report seems clear: existing European health-care systems are unsustainable; fundamental reform inescapable – and, if reform is ducked or delayed, Europe's health-care systems will be seen to fail badly!

The EIU report had concluded that in order to adapt and survive, albeit greatly altered, publicly funded health-care had no real option but to build partnerships with the private heath sector and set strict limits to what they provided. Two factors were said to be critical and of increasing importance to the efficient operation of health-care systems. They were:

- 'New techniques and equipment which allow fast, accurate and effective treatment without the trauma of major surgery'.
- 'Informatics tools for collecting, assessing and communicating outcomes data which allow for improvements in future practice'.

Private versus public

It is far from certain however that either the assessment and use of new technologies in health-care, or the application of telematics to health care confers distinct advantages on the private health sector or undermines the public sector. There are considerable uncertainties surrounding the introduction of new technologies into health-care systems, including the development of telematics applications for health care. Those uncertainties encompass applications and developments that could be highly advantageous to publicly funded health services.

Effective control of the costs and maximisation of the benefits achieved from adopting new technologies in health care are both widely accepted as vitally important to contemporary health care systems (Abel-Smith *et al.*, 1995, xx; Saltman, 1997, 82, 205–6; Stewart, 1999: 65–84). New technologies are said to drive cost increases in health care more strongly than other factors and discriminating between new technologies is not only technically demanding but can quickly turn into an economic and political battlefield. Art Stewart, who has undertaken an international analysis of cost-containment and privatization in health care, has few doubts that *global budgeting*, the ability to act as a single purchaser enjoyed by health care system such as the UK's NHS, is strongly linked to 'control over the diffusion of medical technology' (1999: 73). While 'a variety of methods' are used to discriminate between new health-care technologies 'a strong role for payers' is necessary to regulate their introduction. The European Commission has given its support to the International Society of Technology Assessment in Health Care (ISTAHC). It is an organisation claiming world leadership in 'partnering . . . research and education on the clinical, economic and social implications of health-technologies' (ISTAHC – web brochure: 1). Once again the Commission is to be found endorsing and supporting an international collaboration, with strong academic leadership, built upon specialist knowledge. The ISTAHC is committed to the proposition that the results of independent health-technology assessments should be made available as widely as possible – academically and professionally and, increasingly by electronic means, to the wider community. An alliance, between the Commission, ISTAHC and member states, committed to the social model and the use of the monopsony power that tends to go with it, appears to offer the best route to effective control and dissemination of new health technologies.

We should not forget, however, that new technologies also announce a new age, what might be called an *information age of medicine* – and, quite possibly, an age of medicine without frontiers. Given decisions, in 1998, by the ECJ (in the Decker/Kohll cases C120/95 and C158/96), which supported EU citizens who travelled abroad for the health services they needed (and insisted on the transferability of their social insurance entitlements), basic EU freedoms have become harder to reconcile with the principle of subsidiarity. The rules which govern the SEM and the integration and convergence of telecommunications both imply substantial challenges to the organisation and management of health services, in member states of the EU in the 21st century.

Telematics and the future of health services

Advances in health telematics are inviting more and more *what if* type questions. What if diagnoses, health monitoring, patient consultations and even some forms of surgery were to be routinely undertaken without the need for patient and doctor to be in the same location? What if this were done using *international* databases and expert systems, advanced electronics and bio-monitors, video-conferencing and combinations of virtual reality technology and robotic systems? Anyone who has read accounts of the development of health telematics applications in North America (Viegas and Dunn, 1998) and developed an appreciation of the capabilities of electronic systems (Kaku, 1998) cannot doubt that medicine and telecommunications make a potent combination.

Richard Smith's (1997) account, writing in his role as Editor of the *BMJ*, of a meeting of a diverse group of thinkers about health care in Singapore in 1997, includes a reference to a future scenario 'where new players and transformational technology' flourishes and profoundly alters health care systems. The meeting, arranged by Andersen Consulting, explored many possible futures for health care systems. One future, in which telemedicine had been widely adopted, lead to a world in which health services are 'provided "anywhere", "anytime"'. The hypothecated outcome, for health care, is a world in which '... government [has become] a regulator rather than a provider' and 'industrial age medicine' gives way to 'information age health care'. Cost and the onward march of consumerism, in this view, combine with health telematics and cause the traditional health care pyramid to be inverted, with hospitals and hospital specialists no longer at the top. Jennings *et al.* have developed a model (see Figure 7.2 which is based upon it) that shows health-care

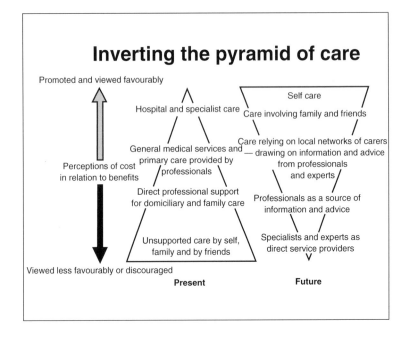

Figure 7.2   Inverting the pyramid of care
Source: Based on K. Jennings, K. Miller and S. Materna (1977), *Changing Health Care*. (Stanta Monica: Knowledge Exchange), as reproduced in Richard Smith, *British Medical Journal*, 1997: 314: 1495 (24 May).

professionals as a resource – facilitators, partners and authorities – available to support self care.

Such images and scenarios invite many questions about telemedicine. Is there any reliable evidence that health telematics represents or will come to represent good value for money? Will telemedicine be able to cross national boundaries when, for example, international co-operation to standardise health data has progressed so slowly? Can health telematics applications pass a CIA test? (de Dombal, 1996: 109). How should *confidentiality, integrity* and *availability* of telematic applications be assured? Aren't enormous medico-legal problems likely to be encountered if health telematic applications are widely accepted? As there are so many different kinds of health related applications possible answers to questions such as these will vary from case to case and from time to time. Steinar Pedersen's (1999) speculations about the future of telemedicine supports a careful *case-by-case* examination of the possibilities. Many kinds of radiological investigation can already be conducted at a distance, using advanced communications technology; 'it is likely [therefore] that ... more and more medical episodes will take place at a distance' (Pedersen, 1999: 191).

More complex and interactive applications will depend on increasing bandwidth – and bandwidth is rapidly being increased. From the patient's perspective remote monitoring of the heart and ready access to individual clinical records, regardless of location, are likely to make some, if not all, aspects of telemedicine very welcome. Pedersen notes that there is evidence of substantial public use of the internet – in the search for medical information. Is it possible that adoption of information technologies at home paves the way for their adoption elsewhere? The ways in which health-care personnel are trained and the division of health care activities between doctors and nurses are likely to be profoundly affected by health telematics. Applications, which enable less expensive health workers to consult more knowledgeable – and costly – colleagues at a distance and in real time, will change perceptions of opportunity costs in health care. There are other questions, however, which it is difficult to even begin to answer. What impact will health telematics have on social inequalities in health and access to health services?

It would, despite the optimism evident in WHO's *A Health Telematics Policy* (1998c) about the benefits and advantages that health telematics can confer, be premature to conclude that the development of health telematics will contribute positively to the development of European health-care systems. Edith Cresson's preface to Paraskevas Caracostas and Ugur Muldur's study (1998) on the future of research and innovation in

Europe, written for the European Commission, also suggests that it is possible to 'marry social objectives with the dynamics of innovation' and to make European societies more economically competitive and innovative without sacrificing the social model (Caracostas and Huldur, 1998: 3–4). The WHO's *health-for-all* strategy assumes that health telematics will become a valued support to policies designed to benefit everyone and generalise access to appropriate and effective health care.

From uncertainty about telemedicine to tackling social exclusion

The political, economic and legal uncertainties surrounding the development, use and regulation of health telematics suggest that the WHO and the EIU are doing their best to influence and shape opinion while waiting, just as anxiously as the rest of us, to see what hatches. Unlike the EIU the WHO has a vision of European health-care policies which stresses the 'fundamental importance of ... socioeconomic prerequisites for health' and promotes the case for health policy to be allied as closely as possible with social and economic policy. The case for concerted European action to tackle social exclusion, in order to improve health, is the subject of Chapter 8.

8
Health, Inequality and Social Exclusion

The most potent and important health issue

Of all the health and health-related issues before the EU inequality in health is the most politically potent. Many social scientists believe that it is also the most important (Townsend *et al.*, 1992b; Levin *et al.*, 1994; Davey-Smith and Ben-Shlomo, 1997). An expanding academic and research literature yokes social and economic inequality together with inequality in health (Blane *et al.*, 1996; Wilkinson, 1996; Gough, 1997: 89–108). The European Commission itself has promoted conferences and publications that advance the view that the EU is as much about improving the life chances and health status of all of the EU's citizens as it is about making Europe more economically successful and competitive. Indeed what could be more important to quality of life than health? Competitiveness is presented as a condition for good health, rather than as the dominant purpose of the Union (CEC, 1994c: 2–3). The need for member state and Commission action to protect and promote health is strongly promoted in Commission documents (CEC, 1997b). Yet the idea that a greater equalisation of the life chances and improved health for European citizens will result, unaided, from the advance of European economies has been widely rejected. With Will Hutton and others leading an intellectual charge in support of more active government and more socially aware capitalism (Hutton, 1995).

Evidence of inequalities in health and attitudes to health inequalities

There is more and more evidence linking a growth in social and in economic inequalities, in the world's most advanced economies, with increasing inequalities in health. Evidence that the *Independent Inquiry into Inequalities in Health*, chaired by Sir Donald Acheson, found was persuasive when it reviewed research findings from around the world for the UK Government in 1997 and 1998 (Acheson, 1998).

Few Europeans believe that their own or their neighbour's life chances should be reliant on unmodified market forces (Abrahamson, 1997: 156–8). Indeed it would be difficult to find a majority in any EU member state to support the view that the chances of living a long and healthy life should be allowed to directly map the distribution of incomes or of wealth. More difficult still, should public policies be thought capable of equalising the chances of living a long and healthy life? Making the distribution of good health more equal than the shares of income going to rich and poor is generally perceived as a good thing and as a job for government. Nevertheless many Europeans (along with their political leaders) also appear to accept, judging by their voting behaviour (and campaign strategies), that the distribution of income and of wealth should be – can only be – driven by market forces. Health policies and social policies contingent on explicit and substantial income redistribution, beyond anything that already occurs, are often viewed as unrealistic. Nevertheless those social scientists, who have the most detailed knowledge and greatest interest in health inequalities, continue to produce arguments and provide convincing evidence to show that social and economic inequalities are the strongest and most pervasive influences on the markedly different patterns of morbidity and mortality being experienced by richer and poorer Europeans (Acheson, 1998: 131–51).

Where might a commitment to greater health equality lead?

Support for a great social purpose, like assuring every child irrespective of his or her home circumstances, a good start in life, may command respect across the EU. Reaching agreement on and building a lasting consensus about the means to achieve such a social purpose requires knowledge and skills, which cannot be commanded in the same way. If health is considered to be a universal good, which citizens are entitled to expect their political leaders to pursue with vision and vigour, political leaders – who are in a position to go beyond articulating the general goal of improving the public health – must expect to be called upon to involve themselves in nearly every branch of government. The breadth of proposals for launching any assault on social inequalities in health can be likened to taking hold of a silk handkerchief proffered by a magician. Political decision makers have good reason to suspect that if they accept a greater role for government, in ameliorating inequalities in health, that it will often be shown – by the magicians with whom they work, epidemiologists and academic health specialists – that their initiatives have failed to take sufficient account of the wider inequalities said to give rise to poorer health and shorter life expectancy in the first place. The uncompromising message from academics and researchers is that health inequalities are knotted together with social and economic inequalities. To tackle inequalities in health you must be prepared to tackle other inequalities (Benzeval *et al.*, 1995).

But direct assaults on economic inequality are highly contentious and raise politically intractable issues for EU member states. EU member states may be co-operators but they are also competitors. And it is not just health specialists who claim that social and economic issues are bound together. Economic policy advisors frequently make the same point and often with a different end in mind. The development of policy in any one area has become increasingly difficult to divorce from any other. Bean and his colleagues, writing about European integration and *Social Europe* argue that: even though the case for harmonisation of social policies has grown stronger, the ability to concert policy developments has weakened (Bean *et al.*, 1998).

It is the interconnectedness of health inequality with social exclusion and economic inequality *and* economic growth that accounts for its political potency and for the considerable difficulties that EU member states encounter as soon as they begin the search for social and economic policies to contain or reduce inequalities. The search for policies capable of reconciling member state's social and economic goals with those of the EU is likely to prove a difficult and frustrating one.

The Acheson report and its implications for public policy

Sir Donald Acheson and his colleagues, in their report on health inequalities for the British Government, illustrated and supported the central theme of their report: pervasive social and economic inequalities are strongly linked to inequalities in health (see Figure 8.1 and Box 8.1). Substantial and growing differences in the material circumstances of Britons were found to exist. Those differences were assessed to have a profound impact on health. And the differences were said to be capable of being modified, in a great many ways, by public policies. If material differences were reduced it was suggested that it was reasonable to expect inequalities in health to be reduced.

The Inquiry adopted what it referred to as the *socio-economic model of health* (Acheson, 1998: 5). Acheson asserted that the socio-economic

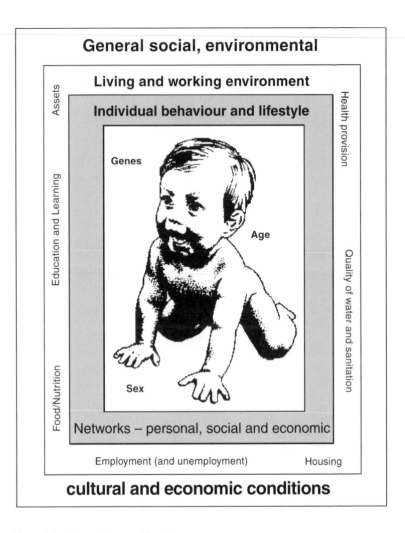

Figure 8.1   Determinants of health
Sources: Based on: Acheson Inquiry Report, Fig. 1 (p. 6) and G. Dahlgren and M. Whitehead (1991) *Policies and Strategies to Promote Social Equity in Health* (Stokholm: Insitute of Future Studies).

model – (which represented the determinants of health status as a complex of interacting layers, including individual life-style and living and working conditions, to which individuals were exposed in different ways, according to their social and economic circumstances) – provided

Box 8.1   Acheson on inequalities in health in England and Wales

- Death rates have been falling among both men and women and across all social groups for the last 20 years but differences in death rates between those at the top and bottom of the social scale have widened. (p. 11)
- In the early 1970s the mortality rate among men of working age was almost twice as high for those in class V (unskilled) compared with those in class I (professional). By the early 1990s, it was almost three times higher. (p. 11)
- Among women the differential in death rates (for women aged 35–64) between those in classes V and IV and those in social classes I and II had increased from 50 per cent to 55 per cent. (p. 11)
- Growing differences in mortality rates between social classes are found across the major causes of death (including heart disease, stroke, lung cancer and respiratory disease). (p. 13)
- Class inequalities in infant mortality remain. In 1994–96, nearly 5 out of every thousand babies born to families in classes I and II died in their first year; the mortality rate was over 7 per thousand for babies born in to families in classes IV and V. (p. 14)
- There is little evidence that the population, taken as a whole, is experiencing less morbidity or disability than 20 years ago; there are substantial socio-economic differences in morbidity rates.
- In 1996, among men aged 45 to 64, 17 per cent of professional men reported a limiting long standing illness compared to 48 per cent of unskilled men. (p. 14)
- Among women (for the same year and same age group) 25 per cent of professional women and 45 per cent of unskilled women reported such a condition. (p. 14)
- Similar patterns emerge from data relating to younger adults, older men and among children.
- Data on obesity and raised blood pressure shows a clear social class gradient among women. 25 per cent of women in social class V are classified as obese compared to 14 per cent of women in class I. 24 per cent of women in class V are classified as hypertensive, compared with 17 per cent of women in class I. (p. 15)
- Amongst men – aged under 55 – major accidents are commoner in the manual classes.

Box 8.1   *continued*

- Mental ill-health and alcohol and drug dependence show striking class differentials. Mental ill-health is diagnosed more frequently among women (aged 16–64) in social classes IV and V compared with women in social classes I and II (24 per cent as against 15 per cent). Among men (aged 16–64) dependence on alcohol was reported in 10 per cent of men in classes IV and V compared with 5 per cent in classes I and II. (p. 16)
- In addition to inequalities in health between socio-economic groups substantial socio-economic inequalities can be demonstrated across a wide range of factors that determine and influence health including education, employment, housing, accidents, transport and health related behaviour. (pp. 16–23)
- The pattern of inequalities between socio-economic groups exists alongside marked inequalities in health between white people and members of ethnic minority groups and between men and women. (pp. 23–4)
- There can be no doubt about the damage that persistent family and childhood poverty does to the health of future generations. (p. 33)

Source:
Acheson (1998).

---

an authoritative and 'scientific' perspective from which to view differences in morbidity and mortality between social groups, men and women, young and old and people from different ethnic backgrounds. The Inquiry Report, which included more than 500 references to academic and other sources supporting its analysis, made 39 detailed recommendations to the British Government (Acheson, 1998: 120–30).

Having demonstrated the close relationship between social and economic inequalities and inequalities in health, in the most objective manner that they could manage, the report's authors concluded that public policy makers had access to a vast policy armoury, upon which they could draw in order to reduce inequalities in health. The message seemed clear, the scientific fruitfulness of the socio-economic model should serve as an inspiration to policy-makers. It should also serve as a warning; no single public policy strategy, to combat social inequalities in health, would suffice. Effective interventions would need to be broadly based and concern with health inequalities would need to shape the whole of economic and social policy. This was a job for the whole of government, not just the NHS. The report asserted that: health inequalities are the outcome of causal chains which run back into . . . the basic structure of society. . . . Policies need to be both *upstream* and *downstream*. (Acheson, 1998: 7) The reference to both *upstream* and *downstream* policies and the distinction made between them by Acheson has considerable significance for the EU and for the European Commission. Upstream policies have a general effect on inequalities and opportunities and are intended to influence social structure and development early in life. Downstream policies are targeted at particular health threats and at those whose health is already thought to have been damaged or about to be damaged. The concepts owe a great deal to the work of J.N. Morris and to arguments he developed in the 1950s and 1960s about the ways in which epidemiological distinctions, between primary, secondary and tertiary prevention, could and should shape public policy (Morris, 1975: 121–41).

A European dimension to Acheson

Even though the Acheson Report was addressed to the British Government it contains numerous recommendations which cannot be implemented without a wholehearted European partnership. It also represents one of the most sophisticated and detailed statements about the relevance of research, on health inequalities, to the whole of public policy that has been produced for an EU member state. The Report refers to 'a wide range of policies' that are needed to 'achieve both a general improvement in health and a greater impact on the less well off' (see Box 8.2), describing them as a response to cross-government issues (1998: 29).

Although this reference to cross-governmental issues was intended as a reference to issues which crossed central government departmental boundaries in the UK it could, with equal justification, be read as a call for international collaboration and co-operation. Clearly in the sights of the Acheson Inquiry team were a number of unambiguously European policy issues with an undoubted impact on health. They were – of course – particularly concerned with the health of the most socially disadvantaged and vulnerable Britons. These Britons were represented as having a good deal in common with their continental neighbours – not least the food policies operated by the European Commission on behalf of the EU.

The cost of basic foodstuffs claims a high proportion of poorer household's incomes. Access to good nutrition is a key factor in good health and particularly significant to poorer households containing children and members with a history of poor health. The *Common*

Box 8.2   Areas of social and economic life covered by Acheson's recommendations

The Acheson Report referred to the need for interventions, to tackle inequalities in health, across a *broad front* (p. 7). Just how broad a front is apparent from a review of the areas of the nation's social and economic life covered by the Acheson Report's recommendations to the UK Government.

- All public policies likely to have a direct or indirect effect on health should be subject to a health impact assessment. (p. 120)
- Social security policies and benefit levels. (p. 120)
- Educational provision and policies. (p. 121)
- Employment policies, including policies that are part of the general economic strategy of the government which can be expected to influence employment opportunities in the UK. (p. 121)
- Housing and environment policies. (p. 122)
- Public policies affecting mobility, transportation and pollution. (p. 122)
- Policies affecting nutrition, including the C.A.P. (p. 123)
- Policies affecting mothers, children and families. (p. 123–4)
- Policies affecting young people and adults of working age (including policies aimed at modifying behaviour – including bringing about reductions in smoking – and encouraging healthier lifestyles – including greater provision of cycle routes). (p. 124)
- Policies affecting older people (including health and social services measures to ensure services are made more accessible to those who need them). (p. 125–6)
- Policies that take account of gender differences (including measures to reduce suicides in young men and measures to improve the psychosocial health of young women and older women living alone). (p. 127–128)
- The National Health Service – its organisation and policies. (p.s 129–30)

Source: Acheson (1998).

Agricultural Policy (CAP) is described by Acheson as a policy that has 'maintained food prices . . . at a higher level than necessary' and resulted in 'the reappearance of food poverty . . . in various parts of Europe including Britain' (1998: 62). The impact of the CAP on the purchasing power and nutrition of the poor takes health analysts well upstream. That did not deter the Inquiry team from recommending 'a comprehensive review of the CAP' focused on health.

Downstream the Inquiry team concentrated its fire on tobacco and the cost of smoking. Without concerted European action and agreement between member states the taxes on goods that are harmful to health cannot be harmonised. Measures to raise prices to discourage 'young people from becoming habitual smokers and encourage adult smokers to quit' will most certainly be frustrated by the SEM if member states do not find better ways to work together. People living in the South of England, for example, cannot fail to be aware of the scale of 'personal' tobacco and alcohol imports. They enable large numbers of Britains, young and old, to avoid UK taxes and duties and to evade the public health intent of UK fiscal measures.

Acheson's net, with or without design, catches other European fish as well. The report makes the case for viewing family friendly employment policies and a strengthening of general employment rights as effective health interventions. It rests its case on evidence drawn from international studies (Acheson,1998: 48). The Inquiry found that British citizens were being denied 'basic employment rights that are a matter of course elsewhere' (Acheson,1998: 48). The development of European regulations affecting the working environment, including the development of parental leave entitlements envisaged under the Social Protocol to the Maastricht Treaty, have become major European social and economic policy issues. While the issues raised are firmly linked by social scientists to health they are – and this is of much greater import politically in the EU – intimately bound up with disagreements between member states about the ways in which social policies interact with and influence economic performance (Meulders and Plasman, 1997: 19–39).

Unemployment and European policy

The Acheson Inquiry team's arguments about the need for government to explore the relationship between the quality of work, the working environment and the health of the poorest citizens, takes us well into EU policy-making territory. They are arguments that need to be considered alongside the Acheson analysis of the damage done by unemployment. Something that takes us to the very heart of contemporary EU policy-making dilemmas. Acheson quotes, approvingly, Richard Smith's view that paid work is 'the glue that keeps our society together' (Smith, 1987; Acheson, 1998: 44). Employment is described as fundamental to the health of 'the population of working age and their families' (Acheson,

1998: 45). Unemployment increases the chances of becoming ill and of dying prematurely and also increases the risks of ill-health being experienced by immediate family members, including children (Acheson,1998: 46–7). Yet the major policy instruments available to European governments, to exert influence over the general level of employment, are subject to ever tightening constraints following the acceptance, by most EU member states, of the disciplines of European Monetary Union (EMU).

If reflationary economic policies are judged to be necessary by health-policy specialists – and recommended by them as a vital part of any plan to improve the health of a nation – it is surely unrealistic for such specialists to expect any EU government to act unilaterally. Health policies, which call for changes in economic policy, appear throughout the pages of the Acheson Report. The political import of the Inquiry's recommendations for European, as well as British policy-making, cannot have been lost on its authors. Talk about the limits imposed on domestic action by economic globalisation and fear of social dumping will always accompany radical proposals, coming from any quarter, to tackle health inequalities.

A thirst for more and for better information about health inequalities

If EU member states have little choice but to work more closely together, in order to combat inequalities in health, they must surely accept and seek to act upon a proposition that is implied or made explicit in almost every recommendation delivered by Acheson. The comprehensive and con-tinuous evaluation of the impact of public policies, in terms of their impact on health and inequalities in health, should become a cornerstone of government action.

The Inquiry team and its Evaluation Group undertook a careful review of a vast academic and research literature on the causes and consequences of inequalities in health. They came to the conclusion that 'controlled intervention studies' capable of informing policy development were 'rare' (Acheson,1998: 29). A continuous *health impact assessment* of 'all policies likely to have a direct or indirect effect on health' was needed (Acheson, 1998: 30). This required, in the words of the Inquiry, 'a significant extension to steps already taken by Government' if government was to be equipped adequately to assess the results of its own policies. The Inquiry team recommended a 'unit with a pan-Government view' (Acheson, 1998: 30). Such a team would be needed to address the fact that the data on health inequality available to the Government was incomplete and lacked consistency. Existing data simply wasn't good enough to monitor the effectiveness of policies or to 'set targets for the reduction of health inequalities' (1998: 30). Acheson – and the Scientific Advisory Group with which he worked – did not seek to disguise the vast amount that still needed to be learnt about the causes and consequences of social inequalities in health and the impact of policies to reduce them.

Margaret Whitehead (1998), author of the *Health Divide* (a key study of health inequalities in the UK) and a member of the Acheson Scientific Advisory Group, has emphasised the extent to which the prospects of developing effective public policies depend on international collaboration. Europe has been described as vast social and economic policy laboratory. The EU is a laboratory that will shortly be considerably enlarged, to take in societies that are significantly different from the established member states. Existing member states vary greatly in the extent to which they have identified health inequalities as a public policy issue. They also vary greatly in the ways in which they have responded to such inequalities.

Sharing information and ideas about social inequalities in health

In an important article on *diffusing ideas on social inequalities in health* Margaret Whitehead argues that:

> the evaluation of policies to tackle inequalities requires the exploita-tion of "natural experiments" that are taking place because of the fact that different policies are operating according to geographic region or point in time.
>
> (1998: 489).

Margaret Whitehead's article offers an account of the growth of interest in health inequalities in EU member states and provides an explanation for the increased political salience of health inequalities. Three EU member states – Sweden, Netherlands and the UK – are surveyed and used to illustrate different ways in which concerns about health inequalities have been mediated by distinctive European polities. The key arguments deployed, in Margaret Whitehead's survey, underline and emphasise the very intimate relationship between the evolution of opinion about the general phenomenon of *social exclusion* and specific concerns about health inequalities. The willingness to accept that broad changes in public policy might be necessary, to combat inequalities in health, is shown to reflect the readiness of those in government to accept evidence of increasing economic inequality. Governments ready to accept such evidence found it easiest to address health inequalities as part of a more general pattern of inequality. In Sweden a change of government and of outlook was quickly reflected in a willingness to consider social and economic initiatives to attack health inequalities. Although Whitehead reports that ideology conditioned policy responses she also concludes that by the late 1990s evidence of growing inequalities had had an impact across the EU on public policy. The facts about health and social inequalities became more and more difficult to resist. The British Conservative government of the mid-1980s is described by Whitehead, as having '[erased] the words "inequalities in health" and "poverty" from the official vocabulary' (1998: 482). The attitude of denial was replaced in the early 1990s, following the departure of Mrs Thatcher from 10 Downing Street, by a reluctant acceptance of data linking health inequalities with economic inequality. Even though some EU member states, such as the UK, were unwilling to embrace research which pointed to a close connection between relative poverty and poor health, both the EU and the Council of Europe recognised the growth of social exclusion and committed themselves and their member states – at least in principle – to containing it and reducing it (CEC, 1998f; CoEPR, 1998).

Social exclusion a pan-European concern

The growth of social exclusion in Europe has been attributed to changes in public policy – as well as demographic and economic change. Perhaps that helps to explain why some EU member state governments have – at times – demonstrated a good deal of nervousness about the kinds of social and health-related research they buy into.

At the same time as evidence of mounting economic inequality in EU member states was emerging (from official statistics and academic studies (JRF, 1995a,b)), attention was also being drawn, by the WHO, to a widening *health gap* between populations in different parts of Europe and within individual European nations (WHO, 1998b: 83). Poor health seemed to go hand-in-hand with social and economic exclusion. The health gap between rich and poor could easily be understood as one measure of a process of economic and social change. A process that was proving damaging for many of Europe's poorest citizens. Particularly – but not exclusively – the poorest people living in Europe's poorest states. Those suggesting that there was a close relationship between material inequalities and poor health could claim, with increasing confidence, that their view had been vindicated.

The impact of evidence and argument about social inequalities in health

Whitehead's account of the diffusion of ideas and information about social inequalities in health has a very special relevance to the work of the European Commission, the members states which it serves and the international bodies with which it collaborates. Her account affords grounds for optimism about the ultimate impact on policy-makers of social statistics on health inequalities and of social scientists' interpretations of them. It also promotes an agenda for international collaborations designed to protect the health of Europe's poorest citizens. Whitehead found that:

- Evidence of deteriorating socio-economic conditions and their impact on health had generated a European debate and influenced the way in which public policies were perceived and discussed.
- Mortality data – showing a widening health gap, between rich and poor, across Europe – had helped to persuade governments and political parties that health inequalities mattered.
- The work of international organisations (specifically the WHO Regional Office for Europe) and researchers concerned with health inequalities had been influential.
- 'The two most striking features of . . . developments [in European research and policy-making had been] . . . the diverse approaches [pursued] and the reinforcing effect of events in one country on the situation in others' (Whitehead, 1998: 487).
- 'Professional advocacy . . . backed by authoritative medical and scientific organizations . . . [had] played [a major part] in pushing national governments to act' (Whitehead, 1998: 487).
- 'European experience [had] shown that, although information alone is not sufficient to trigger action, its availability in the right form can be a powerful tool for advocacy' (Whitehead, 1998: 488)
- Health inequalities are an 'area in which international collaboration can [be expected to] make a valuable contribution in future' (Whithead, 1998, 489)

Whitehead came to the conclusion that the WHO Regional Office had been able to raise awareness of health inequalities and their consequences because WHO had 'helped to create networks of researchers, politicians and policy-makers in Europe to tackle the problem of inequalities in health' (1998: 478). The dissemination of information about health inequalities had enabled and encouraged others, social scientists and journalists, to explore possible relationships between health and topics such as homelessness, unemployment and poverty. This had raised the level of debate and helped to keep health inequalities in the public domain.

Whitehead points to Will Hutton's *The State We're In*, as an example of work which was aided by the publication of data on health inequalities. She implies that data on health inequalities gave a harder edge to the discussion of social divisions in European societies. It led some, who questioned the benefits obtained from shifts in public policy in the 1990s, to formulate better questions (about social inequality) and to look for better ways of getting them answered (Whitehead, 1998: 486). It is clear that, while Margaret Whitehead and other health researchers found they could not avoid *confrontation* with the Conservative administrations led by Mrs Thatcher, it was possible for them to collaborate with academic and scientific colleagues elsewhere in Europe. In that way they were able to help shape a debate about health policy which, eventually, found a government audience at home.

Social exclusion and the social dimension of Europe

The need for a social dimension to Europe, which complements economic development and co-operation between European nations, has been an accepted part of the European project since the establishment the ECSC. Britain's voice of dissent, since joining the EC, heard on almost every occasion when proposals to the strengthen the social dimension of Europe have been advanced by the European Commission, has served to emphasise the broad acceptance afforded by other member states to notions of workers rights and social rights for all European citizens.

In the final decade of the 20th century references to social inclusion and social exclusion, in the documents of the EC/EU and the Council of Europe, have become increasingly common. And, through the 1990s, the European Commission – its DGV in particular – has declared its support for research and social action justified in terms of the need to understand and combat the growth of social exclusion in EU member states. The approach of would be European health and social policy-makers to inequalities in health, that have been forcefully and persuasively presented as a product of increasing economic and social inequality, needs to be understood in the context of mounting concern about the extent of social exclusion and the development of European political rhetoric and Treaty commitments to social progress and social rights. The material presented below is intended to explore both the political context and policy developments which are shaping the EU's response to social exclusion generally and health inequalities in particular.

The Council of Europe – social exclusion a common European concern

The Council of Europe may be dismissed as no more than a talking shop. It has no power to pass legislation but it has, since its establishment in 1949, enunciated standards, agreed between national leaders and parliamentarians drawn from its member states, which have been published in the form of Conventions, Charters or Codes (to which member states can sign up). It is also responsible for issuing Opinions and Recommendations, agreed at the Council of Europe's Parliamentary Assembly. The most important and best known Council of Europe document is the Convention for the Protection of Human Rights and Fundamental Freedoms, drawn up in 1950 and now known as the European Convention on Human Rights (ECHR). The Convention led directly to the establishment of the European Commission on Human Rights and the European Court of Human Rights. The European Social Charter, a counterpart to the ECHR in respect of economic and social rights (often associated with Turin – where it was signed in 1961), is another product of the Council of Europe.

At the end of the 20th Century the membership of the Council of Europe had grown (from 10 states) to provide a forum for parliamentarians from 40 countries (including the Central and Eastern European Countries (CEEC) seeking membership of the EU). Those parliamentarians represent over 770 million people (Bainbridge, 1998: 96–8). The Parliamentary Assembly of the Council of Europe provides a very special opportunity for elected representatives from across Europe to explore major social and economic issues. They can seek out common ground and determine some of the parameters of what might, rather loftily, be described as a pan-European political and jurisprudential family. Ministers from member states make up the membership of a Committee of Ministers, which is the Council of Europe's decision-making body. It is not without significance therefore that the Council of Europe has devoted a growing amount of time and energy to investigating the consequences, for social and economic rights, of economic and social division in Europe.

In January 1999 Council of Europe member state government representatives approved the establishment of a Specialised Unit on Social Cohesion within the Secretariat of the Council of Europe (CoE,

1999). The work of the Unit is intended to build on a European research programme known as the *Human Dignity and Social Exclusion Project* (HDSE). Started in 1995 the HDSE project won plaudits from the Parliamentary Assembly of the Council of Europe (Recommendation 1355 (1998)). It has been described in a Council of Europe Press Release as the:

> The first pan-European effort of its kind . . . [responsible for creating] a network of 17 research correspondents to report on five issues (health, housing, employment, social protection and education) throughout Europe.
>
> (CoE PR, 1997a).

In funding the establishment of a Specialised Unit the 40 member states of the Council of Europe have decided to develop and carry on work begun by the HDSE project. The HDSE project was established to show 'how social exclusion and poverty is affecting the entire continent' (CoE PR, 1997a,b). The Specialised Unit will act on the HDSE action plan for combating social exclusion. The action plan, presented at a major conference held in Helsinki, in May 1998, to set out and debate the HDSE's main conclusions, assumed that the Council of Europe would seek to commit its member states firmly to full implementation of the European Social Charter. In doing so member states would lead an assault on poverty and social exclusion, by strengthening and improving their social welfare systems. They would improve:

- health (by putting greater emphasis on prevention and guarantees of access to health services);
- housing (by building more homes and more affordable homes, responding better to emergencies and taking account of different lifestyles);
- employment opportunities (through commitment to equal opportunities, job creation programmes and sharing out of work);
- social protection (by reforming social security systems so that they were better adapted to contemporary labour markets and helping social workers to become more effective advocates for the socially excluded);
- education (by doing more to combat school failure and the psychological damage it causes and by promoting life long education).

A Council of Europe Press Release, summarising the work and anticipated impact of the Helsinki Conference, reported that:

The Council of Europe has already [responded] to the call . . . to put Social Cohesion to the top of the agenda. A specialised unit is being created to handle social cohesion issues and test drive new methods. There will . . . be a European Social Cohesion Committee to co-ordinate continent wide action . . . and other ideas from Helsinki will feed into future work.

(CoE PR, 1998)

European states – those inside and outside of the EU – could be said to be trying to give effect to commitments made at the 1995 Copenhagen Summit on social development by heads of state and government from around the world (UN, 1995). In the words of a Council of Europe Parliamentary Assembly Recommendation the political leaders of Europe had made a commitment to eradicate poverty through action at national level and through international co-operation (CoE, 1998a).

The EU and social exclusion

Whilst the Council of Europe has been making the case for wider and wholehearted adoption of the European Social Charter the EC/EU has been developing its own policies and approach to social exclusion. It has been trying to find convincing answers to questions about how EU member states can make the European social dimension count without overriding the principle of subsidiarity. The text of the *European Community's Charter of the Fundamental Social Rights of Workers* (adopted by 11 of the 12 member states of the Community at Strasbourg in December 1989) refers specifically to the 'inspiration [to be drawn] from the . . . European Social Charter of the Council of Europe' (Gold, 1993: 222).

The Community's Charter of Fundamental Rights for Workers is an aspirational document, intended to promote the idea that member states would have to act purposefully, collaboratively and resolutely if the benefits of economic prosperity were to be shared fairly. It was also intended to serve as a launch platform for a Commission Action Programme, to integrate member state social policies sufficiently to establish minimum social standards to complement the economic integration being driven by the SEM.

The Commission's Action Programme, published in November, 1989 contained 47 separate initiatives. Almost all of them could have been accommodated within the kind of *broad front* described and recommended by Sir Donald Acheson's Report on Inequalities in Health. The UK

Government had, in 1989, been the only member state to have excluded itself from the Charter of Workers Social Rights.

The text of the Charter became the basis – how confusing the many variations in terminology are – for the Social Chapter. The Social Chapter was intended to be an integral part of the Maastricht Treaty (the TEU). John Major's refusal to accept amendments to the Social Chapter led to an agreement between the other eleven member states to sign up to the Social Chapter in the form of a separate Social Protocol to the Maastricht Treaty (from which Britain was excluded). In June of 1997, following a change of Government in the UK, the UK did sign up to the Social Protocol, its principal provisions having been incorporated into the Treaty of Amsterdam. The Social Protocol is now part of the consolidated Treaties of the EU and applies to all 15 member states of the Union. The Commission has meanwhile sought to build on the Social Action Programme first proposed in 1989 and develop European social action as part of a EU wide assault on social exclusion.

Social exclusion taken more seriously

Christine Cousins in her *Society, Work and Welfare in Europe* explores the origins of EC/EU interest in and involvement with research into poverty and social exclusion (1999: 141–66). The first European anti-poverty programme dates back to 1975. A second and a third programme were in progress between 1986 and 1994. In 1984 the Council of Ministers 'adopted a definition of poverty [that referred to the poor as]. . ."persons whose resources (material, cultural and social) are so limited as to exclude them from the minimum acceptable way of life in the member state in which they live"' (Cousins, 1999: 142). The term social exclusion is now preferred to poverty in EC/EU documents and debate, having been adopted by the EC in 1989, when the Commission was first asked to consider ways of fighting social exclusion by the Council of Ministers. It is a term that embraces many different aspects of social and economic life of which the lack of monetary means is just a part. Cousins, relying on Room, explains:

> The notion of social exclusion . . . focuses on relational issues, that is, 'inadequate social participation, lack of social protection, lack of social integration, lack of power'
> (1999, 145 – quoted from Room, 1991: 105)

Room's definition of social exclusion was echoed in the Commission's own account of a Round Table conference organised by DGV and held in

Brussels in 1999 (Round Table Conference on Social Inclusion, 6–7 May). The conference, attended by some '200 key players from member states and Community level organisations', heard from 'many speakers [who] emphasised the need to affirm a strong political ambition at European level'. To combat social exclusion it was necessary to promote 'an integrated approach, partnership and the involvement of people affected by social exclusion as real stakeholders' (DGV-Commission web site).

However Padraig Flynn, the Commissioner in charge of DGV at the time, had acknowledged several years earlier that the Commission's attempts to secure social cohesion and combat social exclusion had 'often been characterised more by intent than by instrument' (Commision PR, 1997b). A Commission announcement in January 1996 giving details of demonstration projects to be grant aided by the 1995 scheme of *European Funding for Projects Seeking to Overcome Social Exclusion* could not serve better to illustrate the Commissioner's admission that Union declarations ran well ahead of EU action. The Commission press notice referred to Commissioner Flynn's delight at:

> being able to support . . . an excellent range of demonstration projects . . . against exclusion. . . . With 6 million ECU at its disposal, the Commission had been able to aid 85 projects in line with the 1995 budget . . . on poverty and social exclusion. The Commission had actually received just short of 2,000 applications under the scheme, from applicants requesting grants for a total of 260 million ECUs . . . [Commissioner] Flynn explained that 'many excellent projects [could not be funded] . . . because of the limitations on finance available'.
>
> (Commission PR, 1997b).

A call for proposals for work on social exclusion, to be delivered to the Commission before the end of August 1999, made it clear that funds for special initiatives remained limited. Proposals were invited for 'preparatory actions to combat and prevent social exclusion', to start before 31 December 1999. DGV had a budget of Euro 5.5 million to allocate with bidders being asked to find at least 10 per cent of proposal funding in cash from other sources (EC call VP/1999/011).

Social exclusion and the European Employment Strategy

The Commission asserts that its modest spending on 'improving knowledge, developing exchanges of information and best practice, promoting innovative approaches and evaluating experiences' (EC call VP/1999/011) should be set against spending by the ESF and the European Employment Strategy.

When Padraig Flynn gave the Hubert Detremmerie Seminar in March 1999 he could not avoid posing questions to himself about the strength of the commitment of the EU and its member states to addressing the 'phenomena of social exclusion'. He asked 'whether Europe [was] really intent on applying as much political will and practical effort to the employment and social agenda as [it had] to making EMU a reality' (Flynn, 1999). Critics of the EU's approach to combating social exclusion can point to the latest iteration of the European Social Action Programme and suggest that the Union does not takes its own rhetoric about combating social exclusion anything like as seriously as commitments to economic integration and enlargement (Townsend, 1992; Simpson and Walker, 1993: 106–18. CEC, 1998f). In response Padraig Flynn and his fellow Commissioners argue that even though spending on demonstration projects and research initiatives, aimed at combating social exclusion, may be modest substantial EU funds, raised from member states, are being spent on measures, undertaken jointly with member states to improve employment opportunities. Isn't this collaborative effort fundamental to any pro-gramme aiming to combat social exclusion?

In 1995, for example, Ecu5.6 billion was spent on 'trying to help people back into work, on training, counselling and other measures to boost employment' (http://europa.eu.int/pol/socio/info_en.htm). Indeed a mass of information is displayed on the Commission's social affairs web site about the ESF and the European Employment Strategy. Visitors to the web site are told that between 1994 and 1999 the ESF transferred 'a total of Ecu47 billion from the EU budget in order to co-finance actions undertaken by Member States to':

- combat long-term unemployment and exclusion from the labour market;
- develop the professional skills and qualifications of potential job seekers;
- help young unemployed persons to enter the labour market;
- foster the creation of new jobs;
- pre-empt unemployment by adapting workers to industrial change; and,
- improve education and training systems.

Padraig Flynn's case for believing that the EU's ability to combat social exclusion and the consequences of social exclusion is growing and will be strengthened rests on the assertion that European social and economic policies are being tied together by the European Employment Strategy. While the European Employment Strategy assumes government has a part to play the role of member state governments and the Commission is not to be exaggerated. Partnership is the key to the integration of social and economic policy. And integration entails, among other things, governments building stronger partnerships with the private sector and encouraging workers and employers to work more closely together.

Those present on 11 March 1999 at Padraig Flynn's Hubert Detremmerie Seminar presentation heard that the European Employment Strategy had 'four strongly connected . . . pillars' (Flynn, 1999: 6). The first pillar – investment in people to make them more employable (*employability*) – did not require higher spending; what it called for was 'smarter spending'. The second pillar – labelled *entrepreneurship* – relied not on the actions of governments but on individuals and enterprises. The third pillar – labelled *adaptability* – rested on the ability of companies and workforces to build genuine partnerships, capable of seizing new market opportunities and 'harnessing the new technological and economic conditions that are . . . re-aligning production and consumption of goods and services in all corners of Europe' (Flynn, 1999: 7). Government could help but its main role was to encourage and facilitate co-operation between the social partners. The fourth pillar – labelled *equal opportunities* – 'is about mainstreaming equal opportunities for women and men' (Flynn, 1999: 7). Whilst there was a role for legislation and for enforcement enlightened self-interest and a co-operative spirit were of the essence. Co-operation between the social partners – employers, trades unions and their members – was essential.

Action to combat social exclusion – at a modest cost

Like member-state governments, certainly the UK Government, the European Commission appears to be seeking low cost or moderate cost intervention programmes, that can assist and catalyse social change and buttress social and economic policies designed to make enterprises more competitive and labour markets more flexible. Adapting the terminology used in a Council of Europe press release – to describe research into social exclusion – the search is on for researchers and policy innovators who are capable of developing and test driving affordable policies capable of reintegrating individuals and households that have been socially and economically marginalised. Donald Hirsch, for example, has described the United Kingdom as 'searching for a new strategy for protecting the vulnerable in society . . . government wants to promote social welfare and cohesion within tight fiscal constraints, and in ways that encourage active participation . . . rather than passive dependency' (Hirsch, 1997: 3).

No low cost options for combating social exclusion and reducing health inequalities

However the most sophisticated theoretical approaches to health inequalities – based on elaborate comparisons of health and social inequalities in the world's most advanced economies – suggest that governments that are unwilling or unable to countenance extensive income and wealth transfers and substantial changes in the organisation and regulation of employment will be unable to reduce inequalities in health (Blane *et al.*, 1996; Wilkinson, 1996).

In his book – *Unhealthy Societies – the Afflictions of Inequality* – Richard Wilkinson claims to 'bring together a growing body of new evidence to show that life expectancy in different countries is dramatically improved-where income differences are small and society itself more socially cohesive' (1996: 1). Wilkinson and those who have been working closely with him have tried to direct attention to the organisation of human societies, their social and economic structures, and away from the immediate or proximate causes of disease. Given the rate of advance there has been in understanding pathological processes this is not, on the face of it, an easy thing to do. But Wilkinson is adamant that: 'Research has shown us that what matters is the nature of social and economic life.' He is convinced that 'big health differences between societies [cannot be adequately] explained by adding up individual behavioural risk factors such as smoking, exercise and diet' (1996: 2). Richer countries do not necessarily have a healthier population. Differences in living standards between societies are not as important, in explaining differences in expectation of life, as differences in living standards within societies. Most of the citizens of a poorer country have the prospect of a longer life than do citizens of a richer country where social and economic divisions are much greater. There is considerable evidence that the world's wealthier societies have crossed a frontier – known as an *epidemiological transition* – which has greatly lessened, if not eliminated, the health benefits to be obtained for many citizens from increases in income and wealth alone. If the differences between people, rather than their absolute living standards, count for more – beyond this epidemiological transition – then the implications for public policy-makers are profound. Wilkinson suggests that a wholehearted commitment to egalitarianism is a vital qualification for public policy-makers who want to improve the health status of their fellow citizens.

If Wilkinson and his colleagues are correct – once a society has passed beyond the epidemiological transition – making society fairer is the surest route – perhaps the only route – to general health improvement.

Inequality, health and social capital

Wilkinson and his associates argue that it isn't simply the case that material differences count for much less, in societies that have joined the post-industrial club. If the relationship, in the world's most economically developed societies, between society and mortality depends on how equitable a society is perhaps many other health differences, which go unrecorded by registrars of death, have also come to depend on how fair a society is. Wilkinson believes that the evidence that 'the [links] between equity and health [are] largely psychosocial' has become irresistible (1996: 3). Public policy makers should be aware that '. . . the scale of income differences and the condition of a society's social fabric are crucially important determinants of the real subjective quality of life among modern populations' (1996: 3–4). Wilkinson and his colleagues claim that they have been driven, by research evidence, to develop a perspective on health which emphasises the importance of social equity and *social capital.*

What is meant by social capital? Social capital has much more to do with the quality and richness of relationships between human beings than it does with economic exchange; although successful economic transactions may depend on the existence of social capital in the form of trust. Whilst social capital is not to be confused with the economist's notion of human capital it is a stock on which societies can draw and to which they would be well advised to add whenever possible.

Words like love and trust represent qualities in human relationships that exemplify social capital. They refer to aspects of social life which are difficult to put into words but are hugely important to identity and to social intercourse. Social capital is bound up with aspects of human relationships that are typically thought of as being less conditional than the openly instrumental relationships of the market place. Wilkinson draws on the work R.D. Putnam (1995) to help him pin down what it is about communities and societies that leads individuals to behave in ways that suggest a sense of membership and of belonging. Putnam, a student of Italian civic society, describes *social capital* as an attachment to others which sustains the willingness to participate in activities that do not necessarily have an economic or an obvious personal reward. Social capital refers to 'features of social life – networks, norms, and trust – that enable participants to act together more effectively to pursue shared objectives . . . [and it enhances] the co-operation [required] to serve broader interests' (Putnam, 1995: 664–5). Putnam and others have suggested that, as financial capital grows, we run the risk that social capital will drain away. Attachments to one another that have been built upon shared identity and mutual respect will weaken. Such attachments are necessary not only for health but also, ultimately, for the preservation of civil society and for successful economic intercourse and exchange. Such ideas have long been at the core of what is referred to as the European social model. Wilkinson and his colleagues are determined to persuade all those who are ready to listen that health policy, for the 21st century, for societies that have undergone the epidemiological transition, must give priority to sustaining and building social capital. In Wilkinson's own words:

> [If] health is now almost unrelated to measures of economic growth and yet closely related to income distribution . . . priority must be given to the satisfaction of social needs.' (1996: 221).

> Policies on education, employment, industrial structure, taxation and the management of the business cycle must all be assessed in terms of their impact on social justice and social divisions.
>
> (1996: 223)

It is not going too far to suggest that Wilkinson and those who share his analysis believe that the overriding goal of public policy should be to share out the gains from economic growth more fairly. But it will not be possible to scale down economic inequalities dramatically without international co-operation. Anxiety that member states of the EU will soon be engaged in a *race-to-the-bottom* in order to retain or build their share of trade are already widespread (Bean *et al.*, 1998: 79–96). Sharing the material prosperity generated by advanced economies will not, however, be enough. If length of life and, more important still, quality of life, for the majority of citizens in developed economies, is dependent on the stock of social capital ways must be found to make European societies (to employ a term frequently found in Commission documents) more *socially cohesive*. The conclusion, baldly stated, is that economic growth must be subordinated to social growth.

Political economy, social inequality and health policy

Wilkinson's analysis, conclusions and recipes receive support and reinforcement from other social scientists and social commentators. Will Hutton and Tony Atkinson have both contributed to a political economy which urges the reform of capitalism and, in Hutton's case, suggests that more humane and socially responsible capitalism will prove to be more successful in its own terms (1995: 319–26). Hutton directs his most powerful blasts against 'Britain's rather special form of capitalism' (1999, 267). Values and institutions matter. Public-policy makers who want to make Britain a fairer and economically more successful society have to be willing to challenge and change both values and institutions. Hutton puts it rather well: '. . . obligation-less property rights will produce a business culture with a cynical attitude towards taxation, consumers and workers.' (1999: 268) In order to reform capitalism in Britain it will be necessary to change political culture and reform civil society. Individual citizens, particularly Britain's poorest citizens, have to be assured that they matter. Whilst the opportunity to participate economically is vitally important economic and social renewal, which enhances self-confidence and gives citizens greater clout, is even more important. Hutton is suspicious of political leaders, including those with whom it might be thought he has a close affinity, who are unwilling to accept the case for greater equality. Talk of equalising opportunities, rather than promoting equality, signals an 'unwillingness to challenge vested interests' (1999: 256). Saving British capitalism from itself requires the British Government to be much bolder than it has been. In Britain we have a capitalist variant that cannot manage enterprises efficiently and has failed consistently to invest in the home economy. It is even more culpable, for exacerbating social and economic divisions, than the capitalist cultures found in other advanced economies. Hutton's advocacy of a stakeholding society is based on more than an appeal to social justice however. He is confident that a fairer society is bound to be more productive and satisfying for its members. If only the political radicals of the left would make more of the interconnectedness of institutions and values Hutton believes they could do more to influence events and policies. They could begin by initiating a debate about 'a choice of capitalisms, highlighting the degree to which social cohesion and economic efficiency are interdependent' (1999: 268). Hutton claims that:

> Framing contemporary political and economic debates around the notion of stakeholding stresses the values of trust, inclusion, commit-

ment and social cohesion – and demands that neo-conservative notions of the primacy of choice, flexibility, short-term profit-maximisation and fatalism about inequality have at least to be qualified, if not discarded.

(1999: 268)

In similar vein Richard Wilkinson has observed that stressing and promoting social quality does not mean giving up on economic growth. Both Wilkinson and Hutton have a vision of a win–win society based on more enlightened social and economic policies informed by social research:

> the empirical evidence is that the narrower income differentials associated with higher levels of social capital are likely to be beneficial to productivity. Rather than having to choose between equity and growth, it looks as though they have become complementary.
>
> (Wilkinson, 1996: 6)

Atkinson – a case for European action and collaboration

Tony Atkinson (1998), one of Europe's most outstanding academic specialists in the economics of inequality, lecturing on poverty in Europe, has made a powerful case for the EU to play an important role in the fabrication of policies to establish a European minimum income and to combat social exclusion. He begins by quoting the tenth paragraph of the Community Charter of Fundamental Social Rights, adopted by all EC member states except the UK in 1989:

> Every worker of the European Community shall have a right to adequate social protection and shall, whatever his status and whatever the size of the undertaking in which he is employed, enjoy an adequate level of social security benefits. Persons who have been unable either to enter or re-enter the labour market and have no means of subsistence must be able to receive sufficient resources and social assistance in keeping with their particular situation.
>
> (Gold, 1993: 224)

Atkinson examines the case for the EU to *supplement* the activities of member states seeking to protect their own citizens against poverty and social exclusion. He examines the ways in which EU member states might seek to harmonise their efforts and makes a proposal for a European *participation income*.

Atkinson concludes that if the governments of member states do not co-operate over social protection their ability to combat poverty within their own borders will suffer. His principal reason for doubting the ability of member states to combat poverty and social exclusion, on their own, and for dismissing objections to an enhanced role for the EU, on the grounds that it breaches the principle of subsidiarity, may strike the reader as somewhat surprising.

While theoretical risks exist that the poor of Europe will become benefit tourists and member state governments will reduce taxes in a competition – to win investment and employment from each other – Atkinson is sceptical about such developments. He declares that *virtual tax competition* is much more likely than real tax competition. Borrowing Hirschman's (1970) distinction between 'exit' and 'voice' Atkinson describes a political and economic environment in which:

> Workers or companies who perceive that taxes are lower in other member states may not migrate but may seek to exercise political power, or voice, to achieve lower taxes at home. . . . In a world where the presentation of policy, and its reception by markets and the media, are seen to be paramount . . . it may well be that the perceived pressures of virtual tax competition become the most important restrictions on the freedom of national governments to carry out social protection'.
>
> (1998: 145).

The chief justification for a *Europe-wide anti-poverty policy* is to be found in political-economy that recognises and a policy-making community that understands that the modern world is a world of economic and social expectations conditioned and mediated by journalists, market-makers and political actors (including public policy-makers themselves). The power of expectations is not to be denied.

Atkinson's reasoning leads him to support a European minimum income based on a combination of social insurance and citizen's income. The latter would not be unconditional – it would be a citizen's income with participatory conditions. And it would be introduced by member states transforming tax reliefs and allowances into a system of basic payments to their citizens. It would not replace social insurance schemes but would supplement and complement them.

Atkinson's ire is aroused by means-testing and by the growth of means-testing in benefit systems, most especially the British benefit system. He invited the audience, present at his Yrjö Jahnsson Lectures, to consider the unfairness of a means-tested approach to the alleviation of poverty that '. . . penalizes personal effort with marginal tax rates higher than those levied on the rest of the population' (1998: 145). And he called on proponents of basic income schemes to compromise. They should not compromise by giving up their commitment to a basic income for all citizens, without a test of means, or their support for the independence of basic incomes. The compromise required entailed acceptance of a citizenship condition. Such a condition was critical to the political saleability of any basic income proposal. The reasoning was simple: a basic income scheme could only be developed gradually and introduced generally across the whole of Europe if it took account of social expectations. Atkinson declares that he would not pay a basic income to surfers. The qualification for a European citizen's basic income would include:

- work as an employee or as a self-employed person;
- absence from work on grounds of sickness, injury or disability;
- being unemployed but available for work;
- reaching pension age;
- engaging in approved forms of education or training;
- caring for young, elderly or disabled dependants;

Being in or available for conventional employment is not the touchstone for this proposal. The contribution test can be satisfied in a great many different ways, it relies on 'a [wide] definition of social contribution' – but Atkinson is insistent that there must be a contribution (1998: 148).

Health policy across a broad front

If policies for health and health policy are indistinguishable from the broad sweep of social policy and economic policy then proposals, like the one advanced by Atkinson, that call for an extraordinary European collaboration, must be considered to be integral to any worthwhile EU plan to address inequalities in health. As social scientists and social researchers have linked social and economic inequalities more closely to health, they have provided a platform for a great variety of social reformers to advocate public policies which may seem to be remote from health and inequalities in health. Realists, who monitor European integration, will no doubt find plenty of cold water to pour on what is easily characterised as impractical egalitarianism advanced in the name of *better health for all* or *social membership for all.* Charles Bean and his colleagues, who make up the Centre for Economic Policy Research, are well equipped to try and persuade us that it is likely to prove extraordinarily difficult for European institutions to prevent the challenges of European enlargement becoming an excuse for beggar-my-neighbour-policies (Bean *et al.* (1998): 79–96). What place then can there be for EU health policies? But a health policy worth the name, a health policy that tackles health inequalities in member states and across the EU, must be ambitious. European health policy is being moved to the very hub of EU politics even if Europe's political leaders find it hard to understand why health matters, considered peripheral in the past, now take up more of their time and are destined to claim a greater share of their attention in future.

9
Conclusion

Opportunity and realism – the Commission's role

The themes of this book will, by now, be very obvious to the reader and the author's enthusiasm for developing and strengthening European health policy will also be obvious. That enthusiasm should not be mistaken for a belief that the EU and its Commission should attempt to tackle every health problem, address every health issue or try to manage Europe's healthcare systems at a distance. Europe's role is that of a partner – free of many of the responsibilities that go with the day-to-day management of health-care systems. Long may that remain so.

Europe's role and member state expectations of that role (and the work of the Commission in particular) should be founded on a realisation that the Commission is best viewed as a resource and not as a rival. The Commission is and will remain a very small organisation. The Commission has no alternative but to negotiate developments in health policy, through the Council of Ministers, with member states and, since the development of procedures for co-decision, with the European Parliament. Its ability to get things done depends largely on its persuasiveness and its ability to reconcile interests. To be effective – and it needs to be made a good deal more effective – the Commission has to be very clear about where and when it can and should act. This is not necessarily at odds with the view that the Commission needs to be involved across a great range of issues. Involved in many different matters affecting the health of European citizens and the operation of their national health-care systems. The Commission, expressly forbidden from seeking a role in running member-state health-care systems is, nevertheless, able to act as a convenor of meetings, a conduit for ideas and the exchange of experiences. It can also serve as a clearing house for research and as part of an international forum for debate about health and health care systems. It may be justified on special occasions – when there is a clear advantage to be had from doing so – in seeking a role as the author (or more likely the co-author) of new initiatives.

No ordinary broker

One of the Commission's greatest strengths is its ability to link together member state's efforts to improve their health policies. It is no ordinary broker for joint actions and new proposals. That is because it is directly accountable and responsible to member states and, at the same time, an appointed guardian of European laws, regulations and of the common purpose (as set out in European Treaties and interpreted by the ECJ). If member states believe that there is a great deal they can learn from each other and that there are many opportunities to compete constructively and productively with each other then – as an organisation – the Commission is extraordinarily well situated to facilitate competition and shared learning. The Commission is particularly favoured with the resources needed to act as a common instrument to help member states extract maximum benefit from health policy collaborations. European diversity in health care and health policy and, above all else, in social and economic organisation, is a most valuable resource. It needs to be fully exploited. If differences between member states can be better understood and communicated objectively they can help member states to take full advantage of the great diversity and many contrasts to be found in Europe, to improve health policy throughout the EU.

The market and health

The consequences of the SEA – the construction of a SEM – reflect the settled political will of member states to trade with each other on the most open and fairest terms possible. Trade in goods and services, which are part and parcel of modern health-care systems, make up a very considerable part of the SEM. The role of ensuring that the SEM proceeds smoothly inevitably means that the Commission and the ECJ will become involved more and more deeply in setting the parameters for European health-care systems. Refining and enforcing rules, which shape markets in medical technologies and construction work for health-care systems, may be mistaken for interference in member state health services. Such an interpretation would be unreasonable and unfair, when such market regulation is the logical and foreseeable consequence of member state decisions to establish the SEM. The SEM is, after all, intended to expose almost all areas of economic importance in Europe to competition (while ensuring that competition is both fair and safe).

There can be no doubt about the economic importance and relevance to international market rivalries of health-care systems. A partial list of the goods and services required to meet the needs and demands of health care systems is instructive:

- diagnostic equipment used by medical services (from Nuclear Magnetic Resonance scanners to the most basic of laboratory equipment);
- gases and chemical supplies (from those used in anaesthesia to those used in the sterilisation and cleaning of accommodation and equipment);
- design and construction services, used in the building, repair and maintenance of health-care facilities (including hospitals and clinics and primary care premises);
- security systems and equipment (which can be used in many different health service settings and locations);
- vehicles, used for transporting patients (some needing emergency treatment) and supplies;
- computers and other information technology supplies (the hardware and software needed to run the numerous systems used to manage and organise health services);
- telecommunications services (upon which a great many operational health-service activities have come to depend and more are likely to depend in future).

Trade in these goods and services is international and so is the research and development work upon which their improvement and marketability depends. Member states have a common interest in getting the best quality goods and services for their health-care systems and in ensuring that European suppliers can succeed commercially and internationally.

Alan Maynard has pointed out that 'despite the omission of the health care market from the Treaty of Rome, harmonisation in other product and service areas is, *de facto*, leading to the integration of health care policies' (Maynard, 1999: 5). He has also observed that even if the notion of promoting 'free markets' 'is part of the political rhetoric of member states of the EU' markets are 'always and everywhere' the subject of regulation by government and by private organisations. If this is accepted the issue, for health policy-makers and those who wish to influence them, is how markets in goods and services supplied to health-care systems should be regulated. In the SEM that regulation has to be European. The opportunities for defining and pursuing common goals are immense.

The SEM is not only a single market for goods it is also subject to the requirement that it operates in conformity with fundamental European freedoms and safety requirements. Capital and labour markets are to be subjected to uniform disciplines. Maynard invites us to consider the case for generalising re-accreditation requirements for medical practitioners that are favoured in the UK. Should members of the medical profession throughout the Union be subject to the same kind of testing procedures applied to 'Airline pilots [and be] tested every six months to ensure physical and mental fitness'? (Maynard, 1999: 5). If there is a legitimate and overriding concern with the safety of patients and the competence of those who care for them what other safety considerations should shape the Union's regulation of markets. Perhaps the EU should, recognising the potential benefits for health that might flow from greater regulation of food markets, encourage member states to accept new measures. Measures that anticipate and restrict the sale of foods that are known to reduce quality of life not simply those that present an obvious threat to life.

Controls on commerce and regulation of private medicine

A theme in this book, and many others that have been published about the EC and the EU, is the existence of spill overs or linkages between different policy areas. Linkages may be poorly understood or appreciated – especially when new policy proposals emerge or are implemented. There are, however, plenty of people – including knowledgeable academic observers, with a specialist interest in health, who are aware of how one policy leads onto or builds into another. Most are keen to offer their opinion and advice. Economic integration in the EU leads in many different directions and spawns many health and health-related policy proposals. On what grounds can states, which have accepted the case for an ever closer economic union, resist proposals to protect their citizens against private providers of health care who are permitted, indeed encouraged, to offer medical services and compete for business right across the EU? If some providers of private medical services and private medical insurance cover turn out to be incompetent isn't there a case for regulation and standard setting that will apply with equal force throughout the Union? If innovatory pharmaceuticals are subject to evaluation by the EMEA then why not new therapies – especially if those therapies can be purchased privately anywhere in the EU.

Few people expect the Kohll-Decker judgements, by the ECJ, to result in a flood of medical tourists travelling from one EU member state to another for treatment. But unrestricted access to private medical facilities for EU citizens and a gradual growth in cross border patient flows for social insurance/public sector funded services is bound to increase interest in harmonising standards and regulations for the provision of medical services themselves. The requirements of the SEM, already a significant factor in European health policy, will become an even more powerful driving force behind the harmonisation of health service policies in member states.

The precautionary principle, health and the SEM

The application of the precautionary principle – so strongly in evidence in the response to BSE and in the reformulation of the EU's health competence for the Amsterdam Treaty – is set to become more important still. In an open trading system, and against the background of news media that span the member states and speedily transmit information and opinion about new public-health dangers, the EU and its Commission have now located work on public health and consumer protection together in DGXXIV. It would be entirely premature to pass judgement on this reorganisation of work within the Commission but there can be no doubt that it is evidence of the Commission's desire to be seen to act more resolutely upon public concerns about the quality and safety of food.

Health crises and scares – including environmental concerns

In this book the BSE crisis has been considered in some detail. The impact of the BSE crisis upon the EU and upon the work of the Commission has been enormous but its impact needs to be understood as part of a more general phenomenon: member-state uncertainty and perplexity when confronted by risks and uncertainties that transcend national boundaries.

Since the BSE crisis there have been other European alarms, including the *dioxin scare* in Belgium, which suggest that the EU along with its member states remain very unsure about how to respond to health scares. But anxiety about health in Europe is not limited to the uncertainties and risks associated with contaminated foods or the genetic modification of crops. Feeding and responding to anxiety about global climate change and the consequences of technological innovation has become the everyday business of Europe's newspapers, radio and television stations.

If space had permitted an additional chapter on environmental hazards and health could easily have formed part of this book. The themes of risk and uncertainty would have dominated such a chapter. The EU itself supports an agency, based in Copenhagen, the European Environment Agency (EEA), set up in 1993, that has the task of *orchestrating, cross-checking* and *putting to strategic use* 'information of relevance to the protection and improvement of Europe's environment' (EEA mandate EEC Council Regulation (EEC) No. 1210/90). The Executive Director of this European Agency, Domingo Jiménez Beltrán, has made it clear how important human health is to the Agency. He gave the keynote speech at the Third Ministerial Conference on Environment and Health in London, in June 1999. His speech was entitled *'The Environment and Health': Links, Gaps, Actions in Partnership*. Jiménez Beltrán told his audience that: There is increasing evidence that micro-pollutants in food, water, air and consumer products may be causing or aggravating important diseases' (1999). But Jiménez Beltrán also explained that: '... the links between health and the environment are complex ... the extent of public ill-health determined by poor environmental quality is difficult to quantify'. He went on to ask whether the amount of ill-health attributable to poor environmental quality could be as low as 2.5 per cent, a WHO estimate for The Netherlands, or 'as much as 23 per cent all over, as a WHO global estimate shows?' (Jiménez, 1999). Jiménez Beltrán's conclusion, hardly unexpected, was that a great research effort was required in order to come up with informed and useful answers. Like the heads of many other European agencies he does not lack for suggestions about the kinds of research that need to be undertaken. In fact the EEA is expected to 'ensure the supply of objective, reliable and comprehensive information at European level, enabling member states to take the requisite measures to protect their environment' (EEA web site). It is expected to make sure that the European public knows about the state of the environment and that European governments are in a position to assess measures taken to look after the environment.

The EEA is being asked to collect and disseminate high quality information, much of it with substantial relevance to health, not only to member state governments but also in a way that will make it available throughout the EU to its citizens. An important part of its work involves collaborating closely with international organisations in order to 'build synergy and to avoid [duplication of] effort' (EEA web site).

Building a reputation for quality work and for independence, rigour and scientific integrity will be very important for the future of the EEA. However, building such a reputation is unlikely to be a process free of conflict. The funding and support given to European agencies (and, as this book has indicated, there are quite a number of them concerned with health), the ease with which they can work with counterpart organisations in member states and appropriate international bodies, will prove key tests of the strength of the EU's commitment to developing high quality information to inform health policy in the decades ahead.

Developing information and communication systems

The strategies adopted by the EMEA, the EEA, the EASHW – in Bilbao – the EMCDDA and the European Foundation for the Improvement of Living and Working Conditions, all place a great reliance on digital technologies, both for communicating with their member state collaborators, with other European institutions and bodies, and with the European public.

The development and use of ICT is one of the most important themes of this book. It is a great theme for the Commission itself and profoundly important to proposals for the future of the Commission and its work. Work on health is no exception. How can a very small organisation with a very limited number of specialists maximise its impact and cover a vast territory? The intelligent application of digital technologies appears to be the answer to many a European public servant's prayers. Of 43 Commission Green Papers issued since 1993, 13 focus on the development and application of information and communications technologies (using *focus* in a rather restricted sense, because almost all EU Green Papers in recent years refer to the use and relevance of digital technologies).

Green Papers are described by the Commission as 'documents addressed to interested parties, organisations and individuals, who are invited to participate in a process of consultation and debate ... [Green Papers can] provide an impetus for subsequent legislation' (EU Commission Europa web site). The titles of the Green Papers themselves tell an interesting story of attempts by the Commission to add impetus to the processes – commercial, administrative and political – which are bringing about a convergence between new technologies and new forms of governance and intergovernmental collaboration (see Box 9.1).

The Commission has declared that it 'intends to act as a catalyst for initiatives from the private sector, the Member States, regions and cities, particularly through the *Information Society Project Office* (ISPO), whose role [is] to encourage and facilitate the setting up of partnerships for launching applications' (ISPO web site). In the concluding section of

Box 9.1   Commission Green Papers, 1995–98 (with IT an focus)

1998
Radio Spectrum Policy in the Context of European Community Policies such as Telecommunications, Broadcasting, Transport and R&D COM(98)596 final)
Public Sector Information: a Key Resource for Europe – public sector information in the information society (COM(98)585 final)

1997
Convergence of Telecommunications, Media and Information Technology Sectors, and the Implications for Regulation Towards an Information Society Approach (COM997)623)

1996
A Numbering Policy for Telecommunications Services in Europe (COM(96)590)
Living and Working in the Information Society: People First (COM(96)462)
Commercial Communications in the Internal Market – (COM(96)192)
Legal Protection of Encrypted Services in the Internal Market (COM(96)76)

1995
Innovation (COM(95)688)
Copyright and Related Rights in the Information Society (COM(95)382)

1994
Liberalisation of Telecommunications Infrastructure and Cable Television Networks – Part II – A Common Approach to the Provision of Infrastructure for Telecommunications in the European Union (COM994)682)
Communication from the Commission – Green Paper on the liberalisation of Telecommunications Infrastructure and Cable Television Networks: Part One – Principle and Timetable (COM(94)440)
Towards the Personal Communications Environment: Green Paper on a Common Approach in the Field of Mobile and Personal Communications in the European Union (COM(94)145)
Strategy Options to Strengthen the European Programme Industry in the Context of Audiovisual Policy of the European Union (COM(94)96)

Living and Working in the Information Society: People First (CEC, 1996c), entitled 'The Information Society – the European way', it is asserted that:

> The Information Society represents the most fundamental change in our time, with enormous opportunities for society as a whole, but with

risks for individuals and regions. The way we develop it must reflect the ideas and values which have shaped the EU. These ideas and values should be transparent and coherent with social justice [,] in order to win the support of citizens. . . . Improve democracy and social justice by ensuring that the potential of ICTs to provide relevant, up-to-date, information on matters of common interest and to enable citizens to participate in public decision making, are fully supported by governments, with the involvement of non-governmental organisations . . . [and] Reduce bureaucracy and improve the quality and efficiency of public administration at national, regional and local level, and improve the overall benefits of welfare state services, such as health care and education, through efficiency improvements and through the better matching of provisions and individual needs.

(CEC, 1996c: paras 124–5)

Keeping network Europe in perspective

The appeal of what Mark Leonard has described as *Network Europe* is considerable (1999). Leonard's analysis of what is wrong with *Europe* and his recommendations for putting things right rest on re-aligning European politics with digital technologies and what he suggests are more sophisticated and realistic notions of partnership between member states, the EU and its citizens. Leonard believes that the shape and role of the Commission have to be radically recast, if it is to play the catalytic and public service role outlined in several of its Green Papers on the impact and potential of the *Information Society*.

There can be little doubt that the Prodi Commission is looking for a more dynamic role that will put it in closer touch with Europe's citizens. Being able to communicate directly – and clearly – with EU citizens about their health and their safety and being seen to play a valuable enabling role in improving health care and health-care systems, is a very attractive prospect for the Commission. The success of its *Information Society* projects and proposals is critical to making a very public success of Commission work on health and the other EU portfolios for which it is responsible. It would be difficult for the Commission to be leaner – almost everyone agrees that it needs to be made more effective. What Leonard suggests for the Commission is, in many ways, the role that the Commission has been trying to develop and define for itself. Not least in relation to health, where the principle of subsidiarity rules and will continue to rule – OK! What Leonard proposes and urges is a 'single market for government and ideas'. Areas of government, which remain 'national in scope ... but which are of common interest to the EU as a whole', and he identifies *social exclusion* and *health* among these, should be subject to competition, mediated and informed by the Commission. Leonard correctly asserts that '... there will be no support for centralising decision-making', but he is convinced that '... all can benefit from mechanisms for monitoring and peer review' (1999: 40). In terms of the phraseology his recommendations are strikingly similar to the approach identified and advocated by Margaret Whitehead, in her analysis of the *diffusion of ideas on social inequalities in health* (1998). Leonard commends an approach in which:

> Each EU member should see its partners as common learning resources across the full range of policy – so that the European Union becomes a laboratory for policy innovation.
>
> (1999: 40)

Leonard suggests that some of the greatest obstacles to developing Network Europe can be found in the 'mindset' of the Commission and of some member states. He calls on the Commission to abandon its obsession with policy harmonisation and minimum standards. However, the very much greater flexibility he looks for from the Commission will be difficult to deliver without the wholehearted support of member states. And Leonard's enthusiasm for Network Europe needs to be carefully qualified. The Commission needs to be able to employ different horses for different courses. It makes little sense, and it would be at odds with Treaty obligations, to adopt a flexible approach to hazardous substances in the work place or the harmonisation of health data, so that member states could exchange information with each other more efficiently. When Leonard turns to the frustrations engendered by Intergovernmental Conferences (IGCs), billed as the key events for steering the EU and providing it with a clear course, it is much easier to agree with him. The political leaders of member states must shoulder the major responsibility for the appearance of incoherence and for the failure of the EU to identify and prepare the way so that they are able to deal with a manageable set of key issues, at the EU's most significant political meetings.

Leonard's proposals, to tackle the paralysis and ineffectiveness that goes hand in hand with unmanageable agendas and conflicting national interests, require Europe's leaders to find and articulate a European dream that can bind Europe together – in much the same way that 'the American Dream has inspired successive generations ...' (1999: 44). It seems improbable that Europe will find a 'powerful untapped European identity to provide a European dream', which will drive more effective European collaboration. The American Dream looks less and less able to cement American society together. It is this author's view that in the *Information Society* common purpose will have to rest on developing a shared understanding of common social and economic problems and opportunities. Transcendent values and dreams should not be expected to carry a load that cannot be borne by common interests.

The role of the ECJ in the health field

The business of giving a clear expression to shared principles in the EU often falls to the ECJ. Its role and its importance have been another theme in this book. Several ECJ rulings of particular relevance to health policy have been referred to in the course of this book and there is a growing body of case law of relevance to health and health-related issues. The ECJ cases referred to cover a wide range of issues: Heylens C222/86 and Vlasspolou C340/89 [freedom of movement for health professionals and others]; Kohll C120/95 – Decker C158/96 [entitlement to travel abroad for treatment paid for by a social insurance fund]; Merck *v* Primecrown C265/95 [parallel trade in pharmaceuticals and patent rights]; UK Government *v* Commission C180/96 [BSE and the powers of the Commission] (see Hughes, 1992 and McKee *et al.*, 1996, for reviews of European law and health policy up to the mid-1990s).

The ECJ – an extraordinary and serendipitous European institution

Even though the ECJ is often thought of as having focused its attention on trade and trade-related issues it operates across a very broad front and its decisions have made it an increasingly political institution, of growing importance for health policy and health policy-makers throughout the EU. There can be little doubt that it will become more important still. Its independence and ability to make European policy as well as interpret EU law have been the subject of a fascinating academic debate about the sources of authority and political significance of supranational institutions (Kuper, 1998; Sandhotz and Stone Sweet, 1998). The ECJ's ability to advance the cause of '... a certain kind of European Community ... [and] a certain kind of economic integration' (Kuper, 1998: 60) have been examined closely by Stone Sweet and Caporaso. They have conducted a detailed examination of ECJ decisions and have been able to argue persuasively, on the basis of their research, that the ECJ has both a high degree of autonomy from member states, and a strong and distinctive jurisprudential approach. An approach that has given it the capacity to take the lead on a number of occasions, and develop Community policies. The ECJ has driven a role for European law that seems designed to ensure that it accords with and reinforces the fundamental integrationist purposes set out in the Treaty of Rome and developed in subsequent European Treaties.

Richard Kuper, in his *Politics of the European Court of Justice*, reviews the powers of the ECJ and the ways in which they have been exercised (1998). He finds Paul Pierson's (1996) account of the ECJ's growing authority most convincing. The states which set up the ECJ agreed on a supranational body that had sufficient powers to settle disputes between them and to hand down definitive judgements, that could not be challenged or easily changed. There would be little point in having a final arbiter that could not arbitrate conclusively between them. It should not come as a surprise that such a supranational institution sought to entrench its own powers and strengthen its position. That is precisely what the ECJ did. Even though the original signatories to the Treaty of Rome did not set out to create a Court that was supreme in every sphere 'the Court secured the core, constitutional principles of supremacy and direct effect' in the years between 1962 and 1979 (Sandholtz and Stone Sweet, 1998: 101–3). In a series of judgements, that were accepted in member states – albeit with varying degrees of enthusiasm – the ECJ doctrine of supremacy was established. Judges, in member states, found themselves in a position where they had to 'settle conflicts between national law and EC law in favour of the latter' (Sandholtz and Stone Sweet, 1998: 103).

Stone Sweet and Caporaso describe the progress of a partnership encouraged, promoted and developed between member state judges and the ECJ in which member state judges became agents of the ECJ. They also describe a process in which the work of the ECJ came to be dominated not by highly technical disputes between member states or member states and the Commission but by '... references from national judges responding to claims made by private actors' (ibid.: 102). The growth of litigation, involving private actors finding their way to the ECJ, was unanticipated by the original signatories to the Treaty of Rome and many of its consequences have often been unintended. As political and economic integration has progressed the range of litigation which can now, quite properly, find its way to Luxembourg (or be influenced by past ECJ decisions) has grown and so have the ramifications for European policy-making. In its own 'proposals and reflections', *The Future of the Judicial*

Box 9.2   ECJ Cases – 1 January 1990 to 31 December 1998

Court of Justice

	1990	1995	1998
Cases brought	384	415	485
Cases completed	302	287	420
Cases pending	583	619	748
Duration of proceedings (months)			
(a) references for a			
preliminary ruling	17.4	20.5	21.4
(b) direct actions	25.5	17.1	21.0
(c) appeals	–	18.5	20.3

Court of First Instance

	1990	1995	1998
Cases brought	59	253	238
Cases completed	82	265	348
Cases pending	145	616	1008

Source: Appendix to *The Future of the Judicial System of the European Union* (ECJ 1999).

System of the European Union (1999), the ECJ has reported on the growth in the numbers of cases it deals with and in the time it takes to decide them.

There is a very clear pattern in the growth of cases placed before the ECJ. Both the rate of growth in cases under Article 177 (Article 234 in the Consolidated Treaty after Amsterdam) and their origin are shown by Stone Sweet and Caporaso to reflect patterns of intra-EC trade (ibid.: 106–13). More than that the numbers of cases has been changing over time, suggesting a process driven by the real concerns of European enterprises and citizens. Something which member state governments find they are unable to direct and to which they are required to respond. Stone Sweet and Caporaso trace a growth in what they describe as cases concerning *social provisions*. Cases that can be described as supporting a process of *positive integration* (ibid.: 121). In the EU ECJ context positive integration is associated with the development of legal frameworks or 'regimes that replace national ones', whereas negative integration entails the 'removal of barriers to (European) integration' (ibid.: 121). While the impact of the ECJ on law-making that is relevant to health and health-related issues is very uneven and likely to remain so students of European health policy would be well advised to keep a very close eye on the current and future work of the Court.

Social justice, social exclusion and health

The most important theme of this book however is neither the way in which the development of digital communications and networks will impact on health and health policy nor the relevance to health policy of that potent combination – EC-law and the SEM. It is the relationship between health and wealth and the role the EU can play in influencing and mediating that relationship.

A report commissioned from the Henley Centre by the Salvation Army and published at the end of September 1999 has referred to what is undoubtedly the principal conundrum before European public policy-makers as *the paradox of prosperity* (Henley Centre, 1999). Is it any longer possible to make rich European societies happier, healthier and wealthier – all at the same time? While many measures of economic and social progress suggest we are doing better there is also growing evidence that ˙economic prosperity in member states, most notably the UK, is increasingly unequally distributed. Far from being a guarantee of health and happiness the Henley forecasters (and they are not alone in this – see WHO's work on *HFA* (1981) for another example) have produced a report which suggests that welfare organisations will be kept very busy well into the 21st century. The *War Cry* has announced – on the basis of the Henley forecasters' advice – that the battle for social inclusion and social justice is getting tougher and will become tougher still.

The analysis of social and economic conditions and of increasingly unequal shares of wealth and income offered in the Henley report has a great deal in common with the work of Richard Wilkinson and his colleagues discussed in Chapter 8 of this book.

In his Foreword to *The Paradox of Prosperity* a British Labour Party politician, Roy Hattersley, expresses his concern for 'the poor who remain ... surrounded by the affluence of their more fortunate contemporaries', but he appears to miss the main point of the Henley Centre report. It focuses on the consequences of social relativities and inequalities for all Britons – not just the poorest (1999: 5). The 'dwindling' numbers of poor Hattersely refers to are said to remind 'the well-to-do majority that they should not live by bread alone' (ibid.: 5). But *The Paradox of Prosperity* is an account of inequality and social disharmony and of their probable consequences for both the materially well-off and the worst-off *and* all those in between. The report anticipates a future in which the growing wealth gap, the gap between 'the top 10 per cent of people [who] will be 10 times richer than the bottom 10 per cent', has a dramatic affect on almost everyone's quality of life. The threat to the health and well-being of the 80 per cent of the population, in the years up to 2010, who are found in the middle of the income distribution, is as much a part of the Henley Report's account of the future as the well-being of the poorest 10 per cent. Those who are the focus of Hattersley's Foreword. What are referred to as 'life pressures' will grow for most citizens, not just for the poorest. There will be a much greater need for people, from a variety of social and economic circumstances, to 'make private provision for old age'; that includes 'the more than one in five' the Henley Centre forecasts 'will be self-employed by 2010' (ibid.: 6).

Growing incomes are not necessarily good news

The Henley Centre reports that if real household disposable incomes in the UK, in 1998, were to be treated as the equivalent of 100, incomes have risen from 32.7 in 1958. Household incomes, when measured by this index, are projected – by the forecasting Centre – to rise to 135 by 2010 (ibid.: 8). Such growth in household incomes should surely be unqualified good news. Yet surveys of consumer confidence tell a different story. *The Paradox of Prosperity* concludes that 'the economy has now become decoupled from "real life"' (ibid.: 11). Britons don't appear to reflect economic growth and mounting prosperity in their attitudes, as they have done in the past – 'growth has failed to impress consumers' (ibid.: 11). A case, perhaps, of doing better and feeling worse – or, at least, not feeling much better. But it isn't, according to the Henley Centre, simply a case of consumer confidence and economic growth being decoupled. The paradoxical impact of economic growth on human welfare extends much further.

   The Henley Centre, in its report, has sought to persuade the Salvation Army (a task that might be compared to *pushing at an open door*, given the Army's concern with spiritual well-being rather than material success) that economic prosperity is not proving to be a positive influence on perceptions of the quality of life in many areas. For example, it notes that questions about the perception of risk elicit responses suggesting that many Britons feel more vulnerable when it comes to burglary or violence. This is so even though official statistics, about crime and risk of crime, suggest that risks have fallen or are little altered in recent years (ibid.: 12). Among the propositions being advanced is the key one: social cohesion is being lost and social insecurity is growing because material inequalities,

inequalities in life-chances and in the ability to control one's own life are increasing. We are being asked to accept that people who have little in common can more easily come to perceive one another as a threat and that our lives are closely bound together, even when we do not want them to be. As evidence of growing inequality the Henley Centre offers findings from the Joseph Rowntree Foundation (JRF), the London School of Economics (LSE) and the Institute for Fiscal Studies (IFS).

- Income inequality in the UK (mid-1990s) is greater than at any time since the late 1940s (JRF, March 1998)
- A third of British children live in poverty in the late 1990s – three times as many as in the 1970s (LSE, July 1999)
- The richest 10 per cent in the UK receive as much income as the whole of the bottom half of the working population put together (IFS, 1997) (Henley Centre, 1999: 14).

The Henley Centre has also drawn, as this book has, on the work of the Acheson Inquiry, to make the case for believing that growing material inequality is responsible for a growing 'health gap'.

Of course Richard Wilkinson and his colleagues go much further than the Henley Centre. Health in societies that have gone beyond the epidemiological transition is viewed as being increasingly closely tied in with inequality, perceptions of inequality and inequality in the distribution of the social resources needed for self-respect and independent action. The *paradox of prosperity* is that, beyond a certain point, prosperity – having access to more and more material – means less and less. Certainly the good life, for all but a few, depends on being able to satisfy material desires but it depends on much else besides. When there is material plenty an individual's self-worth and happiness – as well as their health – depends less on what they possess and more on who and what they are. Notions of self-worth and the satisfaction of human needs are, in wealthy societies – if Wilkinson's thesis is accepted – more and more significant so far as health is concerned. Social relations and social relativities take on a much great significance – when seeking to explain differences in health. Social differences affect psychosocial well-being and psychosocial well-being is reflected in differential patterns of morbidity and mortality. Psychosocial well-being is – and this is particularly important so far as the makers of public policy are concerned – reflected in the generally poorer expectation of life and poorer health found in rich but unequal societies. This is most apparent when wealthy societies are compared with each other. When the richest societies are compared with other quite possibly less wealthy

236 The European Union and Health

societies, which are more egalitarian and possess a greater stock of social capital.

Once social capital is dissipated it is extremely hard to restore and renew. This proposition is an important part of the reasoning behind Wilkinson's choice of imagery to indicate the nature of the task facing health and public policy-makers. Those who accept his thesis and tie health policy closely to economic and social policy have the job of *putting Humpty-Dumpty together again* (Wilkinson, 1996: 211–32). Wilkinson's grounds for optimism about the task – of renewing and rebuilding social capital and promoting egalitarianism – are also set out in the final chapter of his *Unhealthy Societies* (1996). His optimism rests on three propositions:

- the public appears to be more aware and more willing to listen to arguments about inequalities in health;
- the consequences of very unequal incomes, for example the increased risk of hypothermia amongst the elderly, have motivated elected leaders to change public policy; and,
- there is a growing understanding that the poor health of the poorest members of society is not a matter for the poor alone and has consequences for all of us.

Wilkinson is convinced that the inequalities affecting the poor are part of a way of life, a pattern of life, that affects us all; a way of life that few of us can be satisfied with.

Europe and the future of health policy

The interconnectedness of modern life and the complexity of many of the issues upon which governments are expected to pronounce makes it essential that we try harder to inform and communicate with each other about what we can do individually and collectively to make life better. I have no doubt that we are living in an era of *paradoxical prosperity* and that health is intimately bound up with our sense of personal worth. Health is a product not only of our genes, our behaviour, our physical environment and the material resources available to us, it is also a product of the kind of society we inhabit. The sense we have of our own value is a function of how we live and work together with others. Individuals need to work together – and so do governments – if they are to create the conditions in which it becomes easier and more productive to invest in a better life for us all. The contribution of the EU to health in Europe (and beyond) depends on the EU and its Commission making the most of the new technologies and the plentiful expertise that exists in member states. Europeans have a special opportunity to learn and to apply countless lessons about health and health-care systems and to discover more about the relationships between health and social organisation. Diversity, technology, shared culture and – by international standards – peacefully co-existing states, all help to make that possible. The motivation for member states to give their full support to the common effort that is required to make the best of the world's *most diverse and well connected societies*, to improve health and health services, is obvious. We can achieve much more together than we can alone.

Bibliography

Aaaron, H.J. and Schwartz, W.B. (1984) *The Painful Prescription: Rationing Hospital Care* (Washington, DC: The Brookings Institution).

Abbasi, K. and Herxheimer, A. (1998) 'The European Medicines Evaluation Agency: open to criticism – transparency must be coupled with greater rigour', *British Medical Journal*, 317, 3 October: 898.

Abel-Smith, B. and Mossialos, E. (1995) Editorial, *Eurohealth*, 1 (1), June: 1.

Abel-Smith, B., Figueras, J., Holland, W., Mc Kee, M. and Mossialos, E. (1995) *Choices in Health Policy: an Agenda for the European Union* (Luxembourg: Office for Official Publications of the European Communities).

Abrahamson, P. (1997) 'Combating poverty and social exclusion in Europe' in W. Beck, L. van der Maesen and A. Walker (eds), *The Social Quality of Europe* (Bristol: The Policy Press).

Acheson, Sir Donald (1998) *Independent Inquiry into Inequalities in Health – Report* (London: The Stationery Office).

Ager, B. (1999) 'Development of the Single Market in pharmaceuticals', *Eurohealth*, 5 (1), Spring: 26–8.

Alaszewski, A., Harrison, L. and Manthorpe, J. (eds) (1998) *Risk, Health and Welfare* (Buckingham: Open University Press).

Allbeck, P. (1998) 'Priorities in Public Health', *European Journal of Public Health*, 8 (3): 195–6.

Altenstetter, C. (1994) 'European Union responses to AIDS/HIV and policy networks in the pre-Maastricht era', *Journal of European Public Policy*, 1 (3): 413–40.

Anand, P. (1999) 'Health and risk – an emerging field', *Eurohealth*, 5 (2), Summer: 9–11.

Arrow, K.J. (1963) 'Uncertainty and the welfare economics of medical care', *American Economic Review*, 53: 941–73.

Ashton, J. (ed.) (1992a) *Healthy Cities* (Milton Keynes: Open University Press).

Ashton, J. (1992b) 'Setting the agenda for health in Europe: what the United Kingdom could do with its presidency of the European Community', *British Medical Journal*, 304, 27 June: 1643–44.

Ashton, J. and Seymour, H. (1988) *The New Public Health* (Milton Keynes: Open University Press).

Atkinson, A.B. (1998) *Poverty in Europe* (Oxford: Blackwell).

Baggott, R. (1998) *Health and Health Care in Britain, (2nd edn)* (London: Macmillan).

Bailey, J. (ed.) (1992) *Social Europe* (Harlow: Longman).

Bailey, J. (ed.) (1998) *Social Europe (2nd edn)* (Harlow: Longman).

Bainbridge, T. (1998) *The Penguin Companion to European Union, (2nd edn)* (London: Penguin Books).

Bainbridge, T. with Teasdale, A. (1995) *The Penguin Companion to European Union* (London: Penguin Books).

Bangemann, Dr. M. (1997) 'Completing the single pharmaceutical market', *Eurohealth*, 3 (1), Spring: 22–3.

Banotti, M. (1995) 'Politics and Health', *Eurohealth*, 1 (2), October: 10.

238

Barnes, I. and Barnes, P.M. (1995) *The Enlarged European Union* (Harlow: Longman).

Bate, R. (ed.) (1999) *What Risk? Science, Politics and Public Health* (Oxford: Butterworth-Heinemann).

BBC online (1998a) 'Health: women caught in cancer care lottery', *BBC News Online Web Site*, 29 October (London: BBC http://news.bbc.co.uk/).

BBC online (1998b) 'The woman who discovered BSE', *BBC News Online Web Site*, 19 May October (London: BBC http://news.bbc.co.uk/).

BBC online (1998c) 'The prion: simply mad', *BBC News Online Web Site*, 19 May (London: BBC http://news.bbc.co.uk/).

BBC online (1999a) 'Health: best cancer treatment "a human right"', *BBC News Online Web Site*, 5 February (London: BBC http://news.bbc.co.uk/).

BBC online (1999b) 'Health: doctors furious at longer hours', *BBC News Online Web Site*, 4 May (London: BBC http://news.bbc.co.uk/).

BBC online (1999c) 'Britain's bill for mad cow crisis', *BBC News Online Web Site*, 18 June (London: BBC http://news.bbc.co.uk/).

BBC online (1999d) 'Health: junior doctors face years more toil', *BBC News Online Web Site*, 25 May (London: BBC http://news.bbc.co.uk/).

BBC online (1999e) 'Health: latest news – junior doctors still overworking', *BBC News Online Web Site*, 26 May (London: BBC http://news.bbc.co.uk/).

BBC online (1999f) 'World: Europe – limit on doctor' hours blocked', *BBC News Online Web Site*, 12 May (London: BBC http://news.bbc.co.uk/).

BBC online (1999g) 'Health: CJD deaths could be on the rise', *BBC News Online Web Site*, 21 May (London: BBC http://news.bbc.co.uk/).

BBC online (1999h) 'UK politics: BSE report put back to 2000', *BBC News Online Web Site*, 25 May (London: BBC http://news.bbc.co.uk/).

Bean, C., Bentolila, S., Bertola G. and Dolado, J. (1998) *Social Europe: One for All? (Monitoring European Integration 8)* (London: Centre for Economic Policy Research).

Beck, W., der Maesen, L. and Walker, A. (eds) (1997) *The Social Quality of Europe* (Bristol: The Policy Press).

Beecham, L. (1995) 'Belgian doctor wins fight for training certificate', *British Medical Journal*, 311, 29 July: 282.

Beetham, D. and Lord, C. (1998) *Legitimacy and the EU: Political Dynamics of the European Union* (Harlow: Longman).

Belcher, P. (1995) 'Mr. Allen Larsson, New Director-General of DGV – Interview by Paul Belcher', *Eurohealth*, 1 (3), December: 1–3.

Belcher, P. (1997a) Editorial, 'Amsterdam 1977: New dawn for public health?, *Eurohealth*, 3 (2), Summer: 1–3.

Belcher, P. (1997b), 'Mr. Horst Reichenbach: New Director-General of European Commission DGXXIV – Interview by Paul Belcher, *Eurohealth*, 3 (3), Autumn: 13–14.

Belcher, P. (1998a) 'An interview with Professor Jean-Claude Healy – Head of Telematics Unit at the European Commission DGXIII-C/4', *Eurohealth*, 4 (1), Winter: 10–11.

Belcher, P. (1998b) 'The role of the European Union in health care', *Eurohealth*, 4 (2), Spring: 11–13.

Belcher, P. and Mossialos, E. (1997) 'Health priorities for the European intergovernmental conference', *British Medical Journal*, 314, 7 June: 1637.

Benzeval, M. (1999) 'Tackling inequalities in health: how can we learn what works?', *Eurohealth*, 5 (1), Spring: 29–31.

Benzeval, M. and Judge, K. (1995) 'Time to bridge the health divide', *Eurohealth*, 1 (3), December: 4–5.

Benzeval, M., Judge, K. and Whitehead, M. (1995) *Tackling Inequalities in Health: an Agenda for Action* (London: King's Fund).

Berlin, A. (1992) 'Current trends likely to affect health care in Europe after 1992' in Hermans *et al.*, pp. 3–7.

Berlin, A. and Hunter, W. (1998) 'EU enlargement – the health agenda: public health challenges and opportunities', *Eurohealth*, 4 (6), Special Issue – Winter: 5–7.

Berman, P.C. (1999) 'The impact of the internal market on health systems in member states', *Eurohealth*, 5 (1), Spring: 8–9.

Berwick, D. and Smith, R. (1995) 'Cooperating, not competing, to improve health: the first European forum on quality improvement in health care will provide a way', *British Medical Journal*, 310, 27 May: 1349–50.

Betten, L. and Grief, N. (1998) *EU Law and Human Rights* (Harlow: Longman).

Biaudet, E. (1999) 'Public health at the dawn of a new milliennium', *Eurohealth*, 5 (2), Summer: 1–4.

Birt, C.A., Gunning-Shepers, L., Hayes, A. and Joyce, L. (1997) 'How should public health policy be developed?: a case study in European public health', *Journal of Public Health Medicine*, 19 (3): 262–7.

Blane, D., Brunner, E. and Wilkinson, R. (1996) *Health and Social Organization: Towards a Health Policy for the 21st Century* (London: Routledge).

Bloor, K. and Freemantle, N. (1996a) 'Lessons from international experience in controlling pharmaceutical expenditure – II: influencing doctors', *British Medical Journal*, 312, 15 June: 1525–7.

Bloor, K., Maynard, A. and Freemantle, N. (1996b) 'Lessons from international experience in controlling pharmaceutical expenditure – III: regulating industry', *British Medical Journal*, 313, 6 July: 33–5.

Blotevogel, H.H. and Fielding, A.J. (eds) (1997) *People, Jobs and Mobility in the New Europe* (Chichester: John Wiley).

BMJ (*British Medical Journal*) (1995) 'European Union policy and health: new report leaves much to be desired', *British Medical Journal*, 311, 4 November: 1180–1.

BMJ (*British Medical Journal*) (1996a) 'Focus – Brussels: European Parliament gets ambitious about health', *British Medical Journal*, 312, 27 April: 1060.

BMJ (*British Medical Journal*) (1996b) 'European manpower is predicted to even out', *British Medical Journal*, 313, 19 October: 1012.

BMJ (*British Medical Journal*) (1998) 'Letters – regulating the pharmaceutical industry', *British Medical Journal*, 316, 17 January: 226–9.

BMJ (*British Medical Journal*) (1999) 'Environment and health: Europe's partnerships can be a model', *British Medical Journal*, 318, 19 June: 1635–6.

Bonsanquet, N. (1994) 'The European Medicines Evaluation Agency: the new agency can be an important catalyst for drug innovation in Europe', *British Medical Journal*, 308, 12 February: 430.

Brearly, S. (1992a) 'Specialist medical training and the European Community: is Britain out of line?', *British Medical Journal*, 305, 19 September: 661–2.

Brearly, S. (1992b) 'Medical education', in T. Richards, pp. 30–9.

Brooks, R. with EuroQuol Group (1996) 'EuroQuol: the current state of play', *Health Policy*, 37: 53–72.

Brown, P. and Crompton, R. (eds) (1994) *A New Europe?: Economic Restructuing and Social Exclusion* (London: UCL Press).

Budge, I, Newton, K., McKinley, R.D., Kirchner, E, Urwin, D., Armingeon, K., Müller, Rommel, F., Waller, M., Shugart. M., Nentwich, M., Kuhnle, S., Keman, H., Klingemann, H.D., Wessels, B. and Frank, P. (1997) *The Politics of the New Europe: Atlantic to Urals* (Harlow: Longman).

Burstall, M.L. (1990) *1992 and the Regulation of the Pharmaceutical Industry (IEA Health Series No. 9)* (London: The IEA Health and Welfare Unit).

Bury, J.A. (1998) 'A Future for an EU public health policy?', *Eurohealth*, 4 (4), Autumn: 5–6.

Caracostas, P. and Muldur, U. (1998) *Society, the Endless Frontier: a European Vision of Research and Innovation Policies for the 21st Century* (Luxembourg: Office for Official Publications of the European Communities).

CC Ref. (Commission and Council Reference Documents) (1997) 'Agenda 2000 – Press Release IP/97/660 – Commission publishes its Communication "Agenda 2000: for a stronger and wider Europe" 16 July', *DOC/97/9* (Strasbourg/Brussels).

CEC (Commission of the European Communities) (1978) *The European Community's Social Policy* (Luxembourg: Office for Official Publications of the European Communities).

CEC (Commission of the European Communities) (1989) *The Europe against Cancer Programme: Report on the Implementation of the First Action Plan 1987–1989 (COM(89)185)* (Brussels: European Commission – DGV).

CEC (Commission of the European Communities) (1990) *European File: Europe against Cancer – 1990–1994 Second Action Plan – September 11–12/90* (Luxembourg: Office for Official Publications of the European Communities).

CEC (Commission of the European Communities) – Directorate-General Audiovisual, Information, Communication and Culture (1991) *The Community 1992 and beyond* (Luxembourg: Office for Official Publications of the European Communities).

CEC (Commission of the European Communities (1993a) *Building the Social Dimension: Europe on the Move (Guide Prepared by DG for Audiovisual, Information, Communication and Culture – Publications Unit)* (Luxembourg: Office for Official Publications).

CEC (Commission of the European Communities) (1993b) *Commission Communication on the Framework for Action in the Field of Public Health (COM(93)559 final)* (Brussels: European Commission – DGV).

CEC (Commission of the European Communities) (1993c) *General Framework for Action by the Commission of the European Communities in the Field of Safety, Hygiene and Health Protection at Work 1994–2000 (COM(93)560 final)* (Brussels: European Commission – DGV).

CEC (Commission of the European Communities) (1993d) *The Institutions of the European Community: Europe on the Move (Guide Prepared by DG for Audiovisual, Information, Communication and Culture – Publications Unit)* (Luxembourg: Office for Official Publications).

CEC Commission of the European Communities (1993e) *Communication on the Outlines of an Industrial Policy for the Pharmaceutical Sector (COM(93)718)* (Brussels: European Commission – DGIII).

CEC (Commission of the European Communities) (1994a) *The Budget of the European Union: Europe on the Move (Guide Prepared by DG for Information, Communication, Culture and Audiovisual Media – Publications Unit)* (Luxembourg: Office for Official Publications).

CEC (Commission of the European Communities) (1994b) *The European Union's Cohesion Fund: Europe on the Move (Guide Prepared by DG for Information, Communication, Culture and Audiovisual Media – Publications Unit)* (Luxembourg: Office for Official Publications).

CEC (Commission of the European Communities) (1994c) *Green Paper – European Social Policy: Options for the Union – Summary* (Luxembourg: Office for Official Publications of the European Communities).

CEC (Commission of the European Communities) (1994d) *Communication from the Commission Concerning the Fight against Cancer in the Context of the Framework for Action in the Field of Public Health* and *Proposal for a European Parliament and Council Decision Adopting an Action Plan 1995–1999 to Combat Cancer within the Framework of Action in the Field of Public Health (COM(94)83 final)* (Brussels: European Commission – DGV).

CEC (Commission of the European Communities (1994e) *Communication from the Commission – Community action in the field of drug dependence* and *Proposal for a European Parliament and Council Decision Adopting a Programme of Community Action on the Prevention of Drug Dependence within the Framework for Action in the Field of Public Health (1995–2000) (COM(94)223 final)* (Brussels: European Commission – DGV).

CEC (Commission of the European Communities) (1994f) *Communication from the Commission to the Council and the European Parliament on a European Action Plan to Combat drugs – 1995–1999 (COM(94)234 final)* (Brussels: European Commission – DGV).

CEC (Commission of the European Communities) (1994g) *European Social Policy: A Way Forward for the Union – A White Paper (COM(94)333-July 94)* (Luxembourg: Office for Official Publications of the European Communities).

CEC (Commission of the European Communities) (1994h) *Communication from the Commission Concerning a Community Action Programme on the Prevention of AIDS and Certain Other Communicable Diseases in the Context of the Framework for Action in the Field of Public Health* and *Council Decision Adopting a Programme of Community Action on the Prevention of AIDS and Certain Other Communicable Diseases within the Framework for Action in the Field of Public Health (COM(94)413 final)* (Brussels: European Commission – DGV).

CEC (Commission of the European Communities) (1995a) *Report from the Commission to the Council, the European Parliament and the Economic and Social Committee on the Integration of Health Protection Requirements in Community Policies (COM(95)196 Final)* (Brussels: European Commission – DGV).

CEC (Commission of the European Communities) (1995b) *Report from the Commission to the Council, the European Parliament, the Economic and Social Committee and the Committee of the Regions on the State of Health in the European Community (CEC/V/F/1/LUX/13/95)* (Brussels: European Commission – DGV).

CEC (Commission for the European Communities) (1995c) *Commission Proposal to Establish a Five Year Health Monitoring programme (1997–2001) (Com(95)449 final)* (Brussels: European Comission – DGV).

CEC (Commission of the European Communities) (1996a) *Second report from the Commission to the Council, the European Parliament and the Economic and Social Committee on the Integration of Health Protection Requirements in Community Policies (Com(96)407 final)* (Brussels: European Commission – DGV).

CEC (Commission of the European Communities (1996b) *Proposal for a European Parliament and Council decision Adopting a Programme of Community Action on Health Monitoring in the Context of the Framework for Action in the Field of Public Health (1997–2001) (COM(96)581)* (Brussels: European Commission – DGV).

CEC (Commission of the European Communities) (1996c) *Living and Working in the Information Society: People First (*COM(96)462) (Brussels: European Commission – DGXIII).

CEC (Commission of the European Communities) (1997a) *Intergovernmental Conference Briefing No. 42: Fight against Drugs and the ICG* (Brussels: European Commission – DGIV).

CEC (Commission of the European Communities) (1997b) *Public Health in Europe* (Luxembourg: Office for Official Publications of the European Communities).

CEC (Commission of the European Communities) (1997c) *The State of Women's Health in the European Community: Report from the Commission to the Council, the European Parliament, the Economic and Social Committee and the Committee of the Regions* (Luxembourg: Office for Official Publications of the European Communities).

CEC (Commission of the European Communities (1997d) *Proposal for European Parliament and Council Decision Adopting a Programme of Community Action 1999– 2003 on Rare Diseases in the Context of the Framework for Action in the Field of Public Health (COM(97)225)* (Brussels: European Commission – DGV).

CEC (Commission of the European Communities) (1997e) *Proposal for European Parliament and Council Decision Adopting a Programme of Community Action from 1999 to 2003 on Injury Prevention in the Context of the Framework for Action in the Field of Public Health (Com(97)178)* (Brussels: European Commission – DGV).

CEC (Commission of the European Communities) (1997f) *Proposal for European Parliament and Council Decision Adopting a Programme of Community Action 1999– 2003 on Pollution-related Diseases in the Context of the Framework for Action in the Field of Public Health (COM(97)226)* (Brussels: European Commission – DGV).

CEC (Commission of the European Communities) (1997g) *Communication on the General Principles of Food Law in the EU – Green Paper (COM(97)176) final* (Brussels: European Commission – DGXXIV).

CEC (Commission of the EuropeanCommunities) (1997h) *Communication from the Commission – Consumer Health and Food Safety* (Brussels: European Commission – DGXXIV).

CEC (Commission of the European Communities) (1998a) *Communication from the Commission to the Council, the European Parliament, the Economic and Social Committee and the Committee of the Regions on the Development of Public Health Policy in the European Community (COM(98)230 final)* (Brussels: European Commission – DGV).

CEC (Commission for the European Communities) (1998b) *Guide to the 1997–1998 Telematics Applications Projects*, November (Brussels: European Commission – DGXIII).

CEC (Commission of the European Communities) (1998c) *Commission Communication on the Single Market in Pharmaceuticals (COM(98)588 final)* (Brussels: European Commission – DGIII).

CEC (Commission of the European Communities) (1998d) *Consumer Policy Action Plan 1999–2001 (COM(98)696)* (Brussels: European Commission – DGXXIV).

CEC (Commission of the European Communities) (1998e) *Commission Green Paper – Public Sector Information: A Key Resource for Europe (COM(98)585)* (Brussels: European Commission – DGIII).

CEC (Commission of the European Communities) (1998f) *Social Action Programme 1998–2000 (Com (98)259)* (Brussels: European Commission – DGV).

CEC (Commission of the European Communities) (1999a) *Working in another country of the European Union (Version Available from European Commission Representation in Ireland and on the Commission Irish Web Site – a part of the Information Programme for the European Citizen)* (Dublin: EC Representation in Ireland).

CEC (Commission of the European Communities) (1999b) *Research and Technological Development Activities of the European Union 1999 Annual Report Submitted by the Commission (COM(99)284* (Brussels: European Commission – DGXII).

Chamberlain, M.A. (1998) 'Avoiding, averting and managing crises: a checklist for the future' in S.C. Ratzan, pp. 169–74.

Chambers, G. (1997) 'The European Parliament BSE enquiry: lessons for health policy', *Eurohealth*, 3 (1), Spring: 16–17.

CHCHP (Consumer Health & Consumer Health Protection section of DGXXIV) (1997) *Final Consolidated Report to the Temporary Committee of the European Parliament on the Follow-up of Recommendations on BSE Commission* (Luxembourg: Office for Official Publications of the European Communities). Citizens First Internet web-site: http://citizens.eu.int accessible via *EUROPA* and information for the press at http://citizens.eu.int/en/en/newsitem-6.htm.

Clasen, J. (ed.) (1999) *Comparative Social Policy: Concepts, Theories and Methods* (Oxford: Blackwell).

CoE (Council of Europe) (1998a) *Council of Europe Recommendation 1355 – Fighting Social Exclusion and Strengthening Social Cohesion in Europe – Adopted by the Assembly on 28 January – 5th Sitting* (Strasbourg: Parliamentary Assembly of CoE).

CoE (Council of Europe) (1998b) 'Fighting social exclusion and strengthening social cohesion in Europe (Rapporteur: Mr Gyula Hegyi) – Report', *Doc. 7981 – 12 January*, (Strasbourg: Social, Health and Family Affairs Committee).

CoE (Council of Europe) (1999) *671st Meeting of Minister' Deputies – 19–20 May – Item 6.2 Specialised Unit – Report by Chair of the Rapporteur Group on Social Health Questions (GR-SOC) and Note of Committee of Ministers Decision (CM/Del/DEC(99)657/6.1)* (Strasbourg: Committee of Ministers).

CoE PR (Council of Europe Press Release) (1997a) 'Europe-wide project targets poverty and social exclusion', *Council of Europe Press Service Ref. 202(97)* (Strasbourg).

CoE PR (Council of Europe Press Release) (1997b) 'Colloquy for a Europe that excludes no one', *Council of Europe Press Service Ref. 477(97)* (Strasbourg).

CoE PR (Council of Europe Press Release) (1998) 'Conference draws up blueprint for action against social exclusion', *Council of Europe Press Service (20.05.98)* (Helsinki).

Coghlan, A. (1998) 'Selling the family secrets', *New Scientist*, 5 December.

Coghlan, T. (1996) 'Commision report on the integration of health protection requirements – a response', *Eurohealth*, 2 (4): 6–8.

COI (Central Office of Information) (1975) *Britain in the European Community: Social Policy (COI Reference Pamphlet: 136)* (London: Her Majesty's Stationery Office).

COI (Central Office of Information) (1994) *Aspects of Britain: European Union* (London: Her Majesty's Stationery Office).

Coleman, D. (ed.) (1996) *Europe's Population in the 1990s* (Oxford: Oxford University Press).

Collins, K. (1998) 'The European Parliament's second hearing on the future EU framework for public health', *Eurohealth*, 4 (4), Autumn: 1.

Commission PR (Commission Press Release) (1994) 'Future of the pharmaceutical industry: time to guard against worrying signs', 2 March, IP/94/167.

Commission PR (Commission Press Release) (1995) 'Safety and health at work: adoption of the Fourth Community Programme', 7 July, *IP/95/742* (Brussels).

Commission PR (Commission Press Release) (1996) 'Social exclusion: Commission announces grants for European projects', 23 January, *IP/96/67* (Brussels).

Commission PR (Commission Press Release) (1997a) 'Commission publishes its communication "Agenda 2000: For a stronger and wider Europe"', 16 July, *IP/97/ 660* (Brussels).

Commission PR (Commission Press Release) (1997b) 'Foundations in Partnership: The Example of Social Inclusion in Europe', 19 June, SPEECH/97/141 (The Hague).

Commission PR (Commission Press Release) (1998) 'Public hearing on the future of health policy', 28 October *SPEECH/98/217* (Brussels).

Commission PR (Commission Press Release) (1999a) 'Two new public health programmes for rare diseases and pollution-related illnesses', 23 April, *IP/99/257* (Brussels).

Commission PR (Commission Press Release) (1999b) 'Report on the economic importance of health and safety measures', 22 March, *IP/99/190* (Brussels).

Commission PR (Commission Press Release) (1999c) 'Fight against drugs: the Commission adopts Communications of new EU action plan', 26 May, *IP/99/347* (Brussels).

Commission PR (Commission Press Release) (1999d) 'Speech of Padraig Flynn – European Commissioner with responsibility for Employment and Social Affairs – The new public health policy of the European Union', 29 January, *SPEECH/99/24*.

Commission PR (Commission Press Release) (1999e) 'Green Paper on public-sector information in the information society', 20 January, *IP/99/32*.

Council PR (Council Press Release) (1994) '1823rd Council meeting – Health – 22 December', *PRES/94/277* (Brussels).

Council PR (Council Press Release) (1995a) '1845th Council meeting – Health – 2 June', *PRES/95/161* (Luxembourg).

Council PR (Council Press Release) (1995b) 'Council meeting – Health – 30 November', *PRES/95/344* (Brussels).

Council PR (Council Press Release) (1996a) '1924th Council meeting – Health – 14 May', *PRES/96/132* (Brussels).

Council PR (Council Press Release) (1996b) '1961st Council meeting – Health – 12 November', *PRES/96/314* (Brussels).

Council PR (Council Press Release) (1997a) '2013th Council meeting – Health – Luxembourg, 5 June', *PRES/97/184* (Luxembourg).

Council PR (Council Press Release) (1997b) '2056th Council meeting – Health – Brussels, 4 December', *PRES/97/376* (Brussels).

Council PR (Council Press Release) (1998a) '2086th Council meeting – Health – Luxembourg, 30 April', *PRES/98/113* (Luxembourg).

Council PR (Council Press Release) (1998b) '2131st Council meeting – Health – Brussels, 12 November', *PRES/98/374* (Brussels).

Council PR (Council Press Release) (1999a) 'Agreement on health programmes', *PRES/99/28* (Brussels).

Council PR (Council Press Release (1999b) '2188ʰh Council meeting – health – Luxembourg, 8 June', *PRES/99/185* (Luxembourg).

Cousins, C. (1998) 'Social exclusion in Europe: paradigms of social disadvantage in Germany, Spain, Sweden and the United Kingdom', *Policy and Politics*, 26 (2): 127–46.

Cousins, C. (1999) *Society, Work and Welfare in Europe* (London: Macmillan).

Croxson, B. (1999) *Organisational Costs in the New NHS* (London: Office of Health Economics).

Culpitt, I. (1999) *Social Policy and Risk* (London: Sage).

Cram, L. (1998) 'UK social policy in the European Union context', in N. Ellison and C. Pierson, pp. 260–75.

Danzon, P.M. (1998) 'Competition policy for pharmaceuticals: on-patent vs. off-patent', *Eurohealth*, 4 (2), Spring: 24–6.

Davey-Smith, G. and Ben-Shlomo, Y. (1997) 'Inequalities in health: what is happening and what can be done?', in G. Scally pp. 73–100.

Davidson, M.J.F. (1996) 'ABC of work related disorders: legal aspects', *British Medical Journal*, 313, 2 November: 1136–40.

De Dombal, F.T. (1996) *Medical Informatics: the Essentials* (Oxford: Butterworth-Heinemann).

Defever, M. (1995) 'Health care reforms: the unfinished agenda', *Health Policy*, 34: 1–7.

DfEE (Department for Education and Employment) and DTi (Department for Trade and Industry) (1997) *Europe – Open for Professions* (London: Dti and DfEE).

DGIII-EudraLex (Directorate General III – Industry) http://dg3.eudra.org/site_map.htm EudraLex web site which contains *The Rules Governing Medicinal Products in the European Union – Volumes 1–9* (Brussels).

DGV (Directorate General V – Employment and Social Affairs) web site at http://europa.eu.int/comm/dgs/employment_social_affairs/index _en.htm (Europa).

DGV (Directorate General V – Employment & Social Affairs) (1997a) *Prevention (Special Edition: Tobacco)*, 2.

DGV (Directorate General V – Employment & Social Affairs) (1997b) 'Future Trends in Community Public Health', *Prevention*, 4: 1.

DGV (Directorate General V – Employment & Social Affairs) (1998a) *Prevention*, 4: 2.

DGV (Directorate General V – Employment & Social Affairs) (1998b) *Programme of Community Action on Health Monitoring – Draft Work Programme 1998–1999* (Art. 5.2.b of Decision 1400/97/EC).

DGV (Directorate General V – Employment & Social Affairs) (1999a) *Prevention*, 1.

DGV (Directorate General V – Employment & Social Affairs) (1999b) *Prevention*, 2.

DGV (Directorate General V – Employment & Social Affairs) (1999c) 'Health and Safety at Work – General Presentation' *Europa web site:* http://europa.eu.int/comm/dg05/h&s/intro/genpres.htm (Brussels).

DGXV (Directorate General XV – Internal Market and Financial Services) *Europa web site:* http://europa.eu.int/comm/dg15/en/index.htm (Brussels).

DGXXIVa (Directorate of Health and Consumer Protection [previously Consumer Policy ad Consumer Health Protection]) *Europa web site:* http://europa.eu.int/comm/dg24/ (Brussels).

DGXXIVb (Directorate of Health and Consumer Protection [previously Consumer Policy ad Consumer Health Protection]) *Europa web site – statement of DGXXIV mission:* http://europa.eu.int/comm/dg24/general_info/mission_en.html (Brussels).

DGXXIV (1996) *Bovine Spongiform Encephalopathy (BSE) – Information for consumers – GUIDE – Second edition (GIS-BSE(96)7.5)* (Luxembourg: Office for Official Publications of the European Communities/DGXXIV Consumer Health Section).

Dinan, D. (1994) *An Ever Closer Union?: an Introduction to the European Community* (Boulder: Lynne Rienner Publishers).

Dorling, D. (1997) *Death in Britain – How Local Mortality Rates Have Changed: 1950s–1990s* (York: Joseph Rowntree Foundation).

DoH (Department of Health) (1992) *European Community and Health Policy: Response by the Government to the Third Report from the Health Committee: Session 1991–1992 (Cm 2014)* (London: Her Majesty's Stationery Office).

DoH (Department of Health) (1993) *Hospital Doctors: Training for the Future (The Calman Report)* (London: DoH).

Dobson, F. (1998) 'The UK Presidency of the EU and public health', *Eurohealth*, 4 (1), Winter: 1–2.

Drache, D. and Sullivan, T. (eds) (1999) *Market Limits in Health Reform: Public Success, Private Failure* (London: Routledge).

Dukes, P. (1998) 'The health and medical aspects of the Fifth Framework Research Programme', *Eurohealth*, 4 (1), Winter: 7–9.

Earl-Slater, A. (1997) 'Regulating the price of the UK's drugs: second thoughts after the government's first report', *British Medical Journal*, 314, 1 February: 365.

EASHW (European Agency for Safety and Health at Work) (1997) *Conclusions of the Good Safety and Health Is Good Business for Europe Conference Hosted Jointly by the Luxembourg Presidency of the EU and the EASHW – Bilbao 15 September* (Bilbao: EASHW – access via web site).

EAHSW (European Agency for Health and Safety at Work) (1998a) *Building the Links* (Bilbao: EAHSW).

EAHSW (European Agency for Health and Safety at Work) (1998b) *Priorities and Strategies in Occupational Health and Safety* (Bilbao: EAHSW).

EAHSW (European Agency for Health and Safety at Work) (1998c) *Economic Impact of Occupational Safety and Health in the Member States of the European Union (Report from Thematic Network Group on National Priorities and Programmes)* (Bilbao: EAHSW).

EASHW (European Agency for Safety and Health at Work (1998d) *Proceedings of Joint EU/US Conference on Health and Safety at Work – Luxembourg 13–16 October* (Luxembourg: EASHW – access via web site).

EASHW (European Agency for Safety and Health at Work) (1998e) *Proceedings of the Changing World of Work Conference – Hosted Jointly by the Austrian Presidency of the European Union and the EASHW – Bilbao 19–21 October* (Bilbao: EASHW – access via web site).

EASHW (European Agency for Health and Safety at Work) (1999) *Proceeding of Safety and Health and Employability – Bilbao, 27–29 September* (Bilbao: EASHW – access via web site).

EASHW (European Agency for Safety and Health at Work) *EAHSW web site http://agency.osha.eu.int/* (Bilbao).

ECJ (European Court of Justice) web address: http://curia.eu.int/en/index.htm (Luxembourg).

ECJ (European Court of Justice) (1996) ECJ Press Release No. 58/96, 5 December (Luxembourg).

ECJ (European Court of Justice) (1997) ECJ Press Release No 57/97, 30th September (Luxembourg).

ECJ (European Court of Justice) (1998) Case C-180/96 – judgement delivered on 5 May 1998 (Luxembourg).

ECJ (European Court of Justice) (1999) 'The future of the judicial system of the European Union' (available at ECJ web site).

EEA (European Environment Agency) web address: http://www.eea.eu.int/ (Copenhagen: EEA).

EFILWC (European Foundation for the Improvement of Living and Working Conditions) (1997) *European Working Environment in Figures* (Dublin: EFILWC).

EFILWC (European Foundation for the Improvement of Living and Working Conditions) (1997b) *Working Conditions in the European Union* (Dublin: EFILWC).

EFPIA (European Federation of Pharmaceutical Industries and Associations) (1997) *Second Round Table 'Completing the Single Pharmaceutical Market' – convened by Dr. Martin Bangemann, Member of the European Commission (8 December, Frankfurt am Main, Germany) – Proceedings* (Frankfurt: EFPIA in collaboration with IMS Health and with a grant from the European Commission).

EFPIA (European Federation of Pharmaceutical Industries and Associations) (1998) *Third Round Table 'Completing the Single Pharmaceutical Market' – Convened by Dr. Martin Bangemann, Member of the European Commission (7 December, Paris (La Chapelle en Serval), France) – Proceedings* (Paris: EFPIA in collaboration with IMS Health and with a grant from the European Commission).

EHF (European Health Forum – Gastein) (1999) *Congress Report: Creating a Better Future for Health Care Systems in Europe* [report of the congress held from 30 September to 2 October 1998] (Bad Hofgastein: International Forum Gastein).

EHMA (European Healthcare Management Association) (1994a) *European Union and Health* (Brussels: EHMA).

EHMA (European Healthcare Management Association) (1994b) *Healthcare and European Integration* (Toledo: EHMA).

Eisma, D. (1999) 'How to build a better EU pubic health budget', *Eurohealth*, 5 (1), Spring: 12–13.

El-Agraa, A.M. (ed.) (1998) *The European Union: History, Institutions, Economics and Politics, (5th edn)* (Hemel Hempstead: Prentice Hall).

Ellison, N and Pierson, C. (eds) 1998) *Developments in British Social Policy* (London: Macmillan).

EMCDDAa (European Monitoring Centre for Drugs and Drug Addiction) web site address: http://www.emcdda.org (Lisbon).

EMCDDAb (European Monitoring Centre for Drugs and Drug Addiction) 'EMCDDA Budget 1998' (with links to details of 1996, 1997 and 1999 budgets) at http://www.emcdda.org (Lisbon).

EMCDDA (1996) *1995 Annual Report – Summary & Highlights – 1st Report* (Lisbon: EMCDDA).

EMCDDA (1997) *1997 Annual Report on the State of the Drugs Problem in the European Union (Highlights)* (Lisbon/Luxembourg: EMCDDA – Office for Official Publications of the European Communities).

EMCDDA (1998a) (European Monitoring Centre for Drugs and Drug Addiction) *1998 Annual Report on The state of the Drugs Problem in the European Union* (Lisbon/

Luxembourg: EMCDDA – Office for Official Publications of the European Communities).

EMCDDA PR (European Monitoring Centre for Drugs and Drug Addiction – Press Release (1998b) '"By the turn of the century we must replace ideology with science" says McCaffrey at US-EU Drug Forum', EMCDDA Press Release, 17 July (Lisbon: EMCDDA).

EMCDDA PR (European Monitoring Centre for Drugs and Drug Addiction – Press Release (1998c) 'EMCDDA's 1998 Annual Report: new findings', EMCDDA Press Release, 18 December (Lisbon: EMCDDA).

EMCDDA PR (European Monitoring Centre for Drugs and Drug Addiction – Press Release) (1999) 'EMCDDA informal drugs forum on Draft European Action Plan to Combat Drugs: Gradin highlights role of national drug co-ordinators', EMCDDA Press Release 16 July (Lisbon: EMCDDA)

EMEAa (European Agency for the Evaluation of Medicinal Products) web site address: http://www.eudra.org/emea.html (London).

EMEAb (European Agency for the Evaluation of Medicinal Products) web based general introduction to the Agency – setting out its mission, tasks, procedures and structures: http://www.eudra.org/emea.html (London).

EMEA (European Agency for the Evaluation of Medicinal Products) (1996) *Second General Report 1996* (London: EMEA). [Is available in PDF format from EMEA web site].

EMEA (European Agency for the Evaluation of Medicinal Products) (1997a) 'Statement of principles governing the partnership between the National Competent Authorities and the European Agency for the Evaluation of Medicinal Products – adopted by the Management Board on 4 December 1996', EMEA/MB/013/97.final(EN) (London: EMEA).

EMEA (European Agency for the Evaluation of Medicinal Products) (1997b) 'Work programme for the European Agency for the Evaluation of Medicinal Products in 1997–1998', EMEA/MB/002/97.final (London: EMEA).

EMEA (European Agency for the Evaluation of Medicinal Products) (1997c) *Third General Report 1997* (London: EMEA). [Is available in PDF format from EMEA web site].

EMEA (European Agency for the Evaluation of Medicinal Products) (1998a) *Work Programme for the European Agency for the Evaluation of Medicinal Products in 1998–1999* (London: EMEA).

EMEA (European Agency for the Evaluation of Medicinal Products (1998b) *Fourth General Report 1998* (London: EMEA). [Is available in PDF format from EMEA web site].

EMEA (European Agency for the Evaluation of Medicinal Products) (1999a) 'Work Programme for the European Agency for the Evaluation of Medicinal Products in 1999–2000', EMEA/MB/005/99(EN).final (London: EMEA).

EMEA (European Agency for the Evaluation of Medicinal Products) (1999b) *EMEA Status Report – 25-05-1999* (London: EMEA).

EMEA (European Agency for the Evaluation of Medicinal Products) (1999c) 'Outcome of the third audit meeting of the European marketing authorisation system, chaired by Martin Bangemann – public statement', EMEA/D/MH/8758/99, 22 March (London: EMEA).

EMEA (European Agency for the Evaluation of Medicinal Products) (1999d) *EMEA Open Day 19th March 1999 – from Decision to Market* (London: EMEA).

EP Report (European Parliamentary Report) (1997a) *0020/97 – 7 February (Medina Report)* (Luxembourg: Office for Official Publications of the European Communities).

EP Report (European Parliamentary Report) (1997b) *0362/97 – 14 November (Böge Report)* (Luxembourg: Office for Official Publications of the European Communities).

EP Report (European Parliamentary Report) (1999) *0082/99* February, Page 10 (Luxembourg: Office for Official Publications of the European Communities).

EPS & DGR (European Parliament Secretariat and Directorate-General for Research) *Fact Sheets available at:* http://www.europarl.eu.int/dg4/factsheets/en/info.htm via the Epoque database.

ESC (Economic and Social Committee) (1994) *Opinion of the Economic and Social Committee on the Proposal for a European Parliament and Council Decision Adopting an Action Plan 1995–1999 to Combat Cancer within the Framework for Action in the Field of Public Health (COM(94)83 final)* (Brussels: Economic and Social Committee).

ETHOS (European Telematics Horizontal Observatory) web address: http://www.tagish.com/ethos/ (mirror site).

EU Confirm (European Union Parliamentary Confirmation Hearings) (1999) *Replies to MEP's Questions from Health & Consumer Affairs Commissioner – David Byrne – August* (Luxembourg: Office for Official Publications of the European Communities and Europa Commission Web).

EUPHA (European Public Health Association – web site at http://www.nivel.nl/eupha/) 'Welcome to Prague in 1999' and 'From the EUPHA office', *European Journal of Pubic Health*, 9 (2): 159.

Europa, 'Citizens first' – European Union web site at: http://europa.eu.int/index-en.htm (Europa is the European Union's web server).

European Communities (EC) (1997) *European Union Consolidated Versions of the Treaty on European Union and The Treaty Establishing the European Community* (Luxembourg: Office for Official Publications of the European Communities).

European Observatory on Health Care System web site at http://www.observatory.dk/ (the Observatory has 'hubs' in Copenhagen (WHO Regional Office for Europe), London (LSE and LSH&TM) and Madrid (Escuela Nacional de Sanidad).

European Observatory on Health Care Systems (1999) *Euro Observer – Newsletter of the Observatory on Health Care Systems (Vol. 1, No. 1, January and Vol. 1, No. 2, June)* (Copenhagen: WHO Regional Office for Europe).

EUROSTAT (Statistical Office of the European Communities) (1991) *A Social Portrait of Europe* (Luxembourg: Office for Official Publications of the European Communities).

EUROSTAT (Statistical Office of the European Communities) (1998) *A Social Portrait of Europe* (Luxembourg: Office for Official Publications of the European Communities).

EUROSTAT (News Release) (1998) 'European labour force survey 1997 – over 150 million in the EU have a job – 4 in 10 are women', 14 May, PR No. 36/98 (Luxembourg).

Everest, D. (1999) 'How are decision taken by governments on environmental issues?' in R. Bate (1999.)

Everley, M. (1993) 'EC does it', *Occupational Safety & Health*, April: 38–42.

Farrell, M. and Strang, J. (1992) 'Alcohol and drugs', *British Medical Journal*, 304, 22 February: 489–91.

Ferriman, A. (1999) 'UK proposes 15 year delay for 48 hour week for doctors', *British Medical Journal*, 318, 15 May: 1307.

Figueras, J. and Saltman, R.B. (1998) 'Guest Editorial: Building on comparative experience in health system reform', *European Journal of Public Health*, 8 (2): 99–101.

Financial Times, The (1998) 'Grant pleas for "vital" BSE research turned down in 1991', Back Page: 8 June (London).

Fischer, A. (1999) 'A new public health policy in the European Union – Policy Statement from Andrea Fischer', *Eurohealth*, 5 (1), Spring: 2–4.

Flynn, P. (1995) 'The launch of LSE health: towards a European health policy', *Eurohealth*, 1 (1), June: 13–18.

Flynn, P. (1997) 'The single pharmaceutical market and public health', *Eurohealth*, 3 (1), Spring: 25–6.

Flynn, P. (1998) 'The Future of EU Public Health Policy', *Eurohealth*, 4 (3), Summer: 5–7.

Flynn, P. (1999) *Social Europe after the Euro – The Hubert Detremmerie Seminar*, 11 March (Brussels).

Flynn, T. and Matthews, M. (1998) 'The European Network of Health Promotion Agencies', *Eurohealth*, 4 (5), Winter: 19–21.

Fontaine, P. (1994) *A Citizen's Europe* (Luxembourg: Office for Official Publications of the European Communities).

Freeman, R. (1999) 'Institutions, states and culture: health policy and politics in Europe', in J. Clasen, pp. 80–94.

Freemantle, N. and Bloor, K. (1996) 'Lessons from international experience in controlling pharmaceutical expenditure – I: influencing patients', *British Medical Journal*, 312, 8 June: 1469–71.

Garrity, T. (1993) 'Maastricht Treaty and environmental health', *Environmental Health*, 10 (4), April: 134–6.

George, V. and Taylor-Gooby, P. (1996) *European Welfare Policy: Squaring the Welfare Circle* (London: Macmillan).

Gepkens, A. and Gunning-Schepers, L.J. (1996) 'Interventions to reduce socio-economic health differences: a review of the international literature', *European Journal of Public Health*, 6 (3): 218–26.

Gilmartin, R.V. (1997) 'Balancing innovation, patient needs, and healthcare costs in the European single market for pharmaceuticals', *Eurohealth*, 3 (1), Spring: 29–30.

Glennerster, H. (1995) *British Social Policy Since 1945* (Oxford: Blackwell).

Gobrecht, J. (1999) 'National reactions to Kohll and Decker: synopsis of a German EU Presidency preparatory meeting held in Bonn on November 23–24 1998', *Eurohealth*, 5 (1), Spring: 16–17.

Godlee, F. 'WHO in Europe: does it have a role?', *British Medical Journal*, 310, 11 February: 389–93.

Gold, M. (ed.) (1993) *The Social Dimension: Employment Policy in the European Community* (London: Macmillan).

Goldacre, M. (1998) 'Planning the United Kingdom's medical workforce', *British Medical Journal*, 316, 20 June: 1846–47.

Gogl, A. (1998) 'Health and enlargement of the EU: views of a candidate country', *Eurohealth*, 4 (4), Autumn: 17–18.

Gouvras, G. (1999) 'Application of risk assessment and management in EU policies and measures', *Eurohealth*, 5 (2), Summer: 19–20.

Gouvras, G. and Delaney, F.M. (1997) 'The Dutch Presidency and the health Interests of the European citizen', *Eurohealth*, 3 (2), Summer: 15–16.

Gore, A. (1992) *Earth in the Balance: Forging a New Common Purpose* (London: Earthscan).

Gott, M. for the European Foundation for the Improvement of Living and Working Conditions (1995) *Telematics for Health: the Role of Telehealth and Telemedicine in Homes and Communities* (Luxembourg: Office for Official Publications of the European Communities with Radcliffe Medical Press).

Gough, I. (1997) 'Social aspects of the European model and its economic consequences' in W. Beck *et al.*, pp. 89–108.

Grant, W. (1997) 'BSE and the politics of food' in P. Dunleavey *et al.* (eds) *Developments in British Politics 5* (London: Macmillan).

Green, D.G. (1987) *Medicines in the Marketplace: a Study of Safety Regulation and Price Control in the Supply of Prescription Medicines (IEA Health Unit Paper No. 1)* (London: The IEA Health Unit).

Greenberg, M.R., Sandman, P.M., Sachsman, D.B. and Salomone, K.L. (1988) 'Network television news coverage of environmental risks', *Environment*, 31 (2): 16–20, 40–4.

Greenwood, J. (1997) *Representing Interests in the European Union* (London: Macmillan).

Griffiths, S. and Hunter, D.J. (eds) (1999) *Perspectives in Public Health* (Abingdon: Radcliffe Medical Press).

Hall, C. (1995) 'UK "failing in diagnosis of cancer patients"', *Independent*, 17 May.

Ham, C. (1992) 'The European Community and UK health' and health services', in A. Harrison with S. Bruscini, (pp. 138–41.)

Ham, C. (ed.) (1997) *Health Care Reform: Learning from International Experience* (Buckingham: Open University Press).

Ham, C. and Berman, P. (1992) 'Health policy in Europe: many changes will result from new chapter on public health', *British Medical Journal*, 304, 4 April: 855–6.

Hantrais, L. (1995) *Social Policy in the European Union* (London: Macmillan).

Harrison, A. (ed.) (1997) Health Care UK: 1996/97 – the King's Fund Annual Review of Health Policy (London: King's Fund Institute).

Harrison, A. with Bruscini, S. (1992) *Health Care UK: 1991 – an Annual Review of Health Care Policy* (London: King's Fund Institute).

Hayes, A. (1998) 'The EU and Public Health Beyond the Year 2000', *Eurohealth*, 4 (4), Autumn: 2–4.

HEA (Health Education Authority) (1995) *Investing in Health – Annual Report 1994/ 1995* (London: Health Education Authority).

Healy, J-C. (Chairman) (1997) *Report of the Strategic Requirements Board (Telematics Applications Programme – Sector Health Care)* (Brussels: European Commission DGXIII).

Hebenton, B. and Thomas, T. (1992) 'Rocky path to Europol: Europe's police see information-sharing as the key to controlling the traffickers, but who controls the controllers?', *Druglink*, Nov./Dec.: 8–10.

Henig, S. (1997) *The Uniting of Europe: from Discord to Concord* (London: Routledge).

Henley Centre (1999) *The Paradox of Prosperity* (London: Salvation Army).

Hermans, H.E.G.M. (1997) 'Patients' rights in the European Union: cross-border care as an example of the right to health', *European Journal of Public Health*, 7 (3) Supplement: 11–17.

Hermans, H.E.G.M., Casparie, A.F. and Paelinck, J.H.P. (eds) (1992) *Health Care in Europe after 1992* (Aldershot: Dartmouth).

Hermesse, J., Lewalle, H. and Palm, W. (1997) 'Patient mobility within the European Union', *European Journal of Public Health*, 7 (3) Supplement: 4–10.

Hervey, T. (1998) *European Social Law and Policy* (Harlow: Longman).

Herxheimer, A. (1996) 'The European Medicines Evaluation Agency: moving towards more transparent drug registration systems', *British Medical Journal*, 312, 17 February: 394.

Herxheimer, A. (1999) 'Towards the Single Market in pharmaceuticals: DGIII's hopes and suggestions', *Eurohealth*, 5 (1), Spring: 25–6.

Hine, D. and Hussein, K. (eds) (1998) *Beyond the Market: the EU and National Social Policy* (London: Routledge).

Hirsch, D. (ed.) (1997) *Social Protection and Inclusion: European Challenges for the United Kingdom* (York: Joseph Rowntree Foundation).

Hirsch, F (1977) *Social Limits to Growth* (London: Routledge & Kegan Paul).

Hirschman, A.O. (1970) *Exit, Voice and Loyalty: Responses to Decline in Firms, Organizations and States* (Cambridge, Massachusetts: Harvard University Press).

HoC (House of Commons) Health Committee (1992) *Third Report 1991–1992 – The European Community and Health Policy (Report together with Appendix, the Proceedings of the Committee, Minutes of Evidence and Appendices) HC 180* (London: Her Majesty's Stationery Office).

Holland, W. (1999) 'Inequalities in health – commentary by Walter W. Holland', *Eurohealth*, 5 (1), Spring: 35–6.

Holm, L. and Smidt, S. (1997) 'Uncovering social structures and status differences in health systems', *European Journal of Public Health*, 7 (4): 373–8.

Hope, J. (1999) 'Britain bottom of the health league' and 'Sick at heart, our NHS: Britain's Third World wards', *Daily Mail*, 13 August: 1, 4–5.

HPM (Healthcare Parliamentary Monitor) (1999) 'Private healthcare in the EU faces "explosive growth": Economist Intelligence Unit report on expansion in the next decade', *Healthcare Parliamentary Monitor* – Issue No. 236 (26 July) (London: Cadmus Newsletters).

Hübel, M. (1998) 'Evaluating the health impact of policies: a challenge', *Eurohealth*, 4 (3), Summer: 27–9.

Hunt, W.J. (1998) 'European Union and public health: a time for debate', *Eurohealth*, 4 (3), Summer: 1.

Hughes, C. (1992) 'European law, medicine, and the social charter', *British Medical Journal*, 304, 14 March: 700–3.

Hunter, D.J. (1998) 'Managing the public's health', *Eurohealth*, 4 (3), Summer: 39–41.

Hunter, W. (1997) 'Future trends in public health', *Eurohealth*, 3 (2), Summer: 12–14.

Hunter, W. and Hübel, M. (1996) 'Integration of health protection requirements into European Community policies', *Eurohealth*, 2 (4): 4–5.

Hutton, W. (1995) *The State We're in* (London: Jonathan Cape).

Hutton, W. (1999) *The Stakeholding Society: Writings on Politics and Economics,* edited by David Goldblatt (Cambridge: Polity Press in association with Basil Blackwell).

Huttunen, J. (1999) 'Contribution of research to European public health policy', *Eurohealth*, 5 (1), Spring: 9–10.

Iakovidis, I. (1998) 'Health telematics: 10 years of European research and Development', *Eurohealth*, 4 (1), Winter: 11–13.

IGC (Intergovernmental Conference) (1997) *IGC Briefing No. 42 – March* (Brussels: European Commission).

IMS International (1996) *Round Table [One] 'Completing the Single Pharmaceutical Market' – Convened by Dr. Martin Bagemann, Member of the European Commission (9 December – Frankfurt am Main, Germany) – Proceedings* (Frankfurt am Main: IMS International in association with EFPIA and Pharmaceutical Partners for Better Health Care).

ISPO (Information Society Project Office) web site address: http://www.ispo.cec.be/ (Brussels-Luxembourg: Information Society Project Office).

ISTAHC (International Society of Technology Assessment in Health Care) web address: http://painkeep.hbesoftware.com/istahc/index.html (Home Page).

Jackson, C. (1995) 'European Public Health Policy', *Eurohealth*, 1 (2), October: 11–14.

Jakubowski, E. and Busse, R. with Chambers, R. (1998) *Health Care Systems in the EU: a Comparative Study – Directorate General for Research Working Paper for the European Parliament [Public Health and Consumer Protection Series – SACO 101 EN]* (Luxembourg: European Parliament).

James, P. (1993) 'Occupational Health and Safety' in M. Gold, (135–52.)

Jencks, S. and Schieber, G. (1991) 'Containing health care costs: what bullet to bite?', *Health Care Financing Review Annual Supplement*, 1–12.

JESP Digest (Journal of European Social Policy Digest) (1997) 'Part 4 – Public health', *Journal of European Social Policy*, 7 (3): 259–60, 263–4.

JESP Digest (Journal of European Social Policy Digest) (1998a) 'Part 3 – Public health', *Journal of European Social Policy*, 8 (1): 83–85, 91.

JESP Digest (Journal of European Social Policy Digest) (1998b) 'Part 7 – Public health', *Journal of European Social Policy*, 8 (2): 182–184, 186.

JESP Digest (Journal of European Social Policy Digest) (1998c) ' Part 7 – Public health', *Journal of European Social Policy*, 8 (3): 260–1.

JESP Digest (Journal of European Social Policy Digest) (1998d) 'Part 8 – Public health', *Journal of European Social Policy*, 8 (4): 337–8.

JESP Digest (Journal of European Social Policy Digest) (1999a) 'Part 8 – Public health', *Journal of European Social Policy*, 9 (1): 85–7.

JESP Digest (Journal of European Social Policy Digest) 1999b) 'Part 8 – Public Health', *Journal of European Social Policy*, 9 (2): 183–5.

Jiménez Beltrán, D. (1999) 'The environment and health: links, gaps, actions in partnership', Third Ministerial Conference on Environment and Health London, 16 June (Copenhagen: European Environment Agency – web site).

Joffe, M. (1996) 'Health and other European policy areas', *Eurohealth*, 2 (2), June: 21–2.

Johnson, T., Larkin, G. and Saks, M. (eds) (1995) *Health Professions and the State in Europe* (Routledge: London)

Jowell, T. (1997) 'Future public health agenda for Europe', *Eurohealth*, 3 (3), Autumn: 11–12.

Jowell, T. (1998) 'Developing EU public health policy', *Eurohealth*, 4 (3), Summer: 2–5.

JRF (Joseph Rowntree Foundation) (1995a) *Joseph Rowntree Foundation Inquiry into Income and Wealth, Vol. 1* (chaired by Sir Peter Barclay) (York: Joseph Rowntree Foundation).

JRF (Joseph Rowntree Foundation) (1995b) *Joseph Rowntree Foundation Inquiry into Income and Wealth, Vol. 2: a Summary of the Evidence,* (by John Hills) (York: Joseph Rowntree Foundation).

Jukes, G. (1999) 'Environmental health perspectives' in S. Griffiths and D.J. Hunter (pp. 198–202.)

Kaku, M. (1998) *Visions: How Science Will Revolutionize the Twenty-First Century* (Oxford: Oxford University Press).

Kalra, D. (1994) 'Electronic health records: the European scene', *British Medical Journal*, 309, 19 November: 1358–61.

Kanavos, P. (1999) 'Health as a tradable service: a prospective view of the European Union', *Eurohealth*, 5 (1), Spring: 18–20.

Kapteyn, P.J.G., Verloren van Themaat, P. and Gormley, L.W. (1998) *Introduction to the Law of the European Communities*, 3rd edn edited and further revised by Laurence W. Gormley (London: Kluwer Law International).

Keck, J. (1999) 'The European Union single market in pharmaceuticals', *Eurohealth*, 5 (1), Spring: 23–5.

Klemperer, F. (1996) 'How to do it: work in the European Union', *British Medical Journal*, 312, 2 March: 567–70.

Kuper, R. (1998) *The Politics of the European Court of Justice* (London: Kogan Page).

Lahelma, E. and Arber, S. (1994) 'Health inequalities among men and women in contrasting welfare states: Britain and three Nordic countries compared', *European Journal of Public Health*, 4 (3): 213–26.

Lahure, J. (1997) 'Public health in the European Union under the Luxembourg Presidency', *Eurohealth*, 3 (2), Summer: 9–11.

Lang, T. (1998) 'BSE and CJD: recent developments' in T. Ratzan, pp. 65–85.

Lefebvre, A. (1998) 'The future of European health policy', *Eurohealth*, 4 (5): 2–3.

Leibfried, S. (1994) 'The social dimension of the European Union: en route to positively joint sovereignty?', *Journal of European Social Policy*, 4 (4): 239–62.

Leibfried, S. and Pierson, P. (eds) (1995) *European Social Policy: Between Fragmentation and Integration* (Washington, DC: The Brookings Institution).

Leonard, M. (1999) *Network Europe: the New Case for Europe* (London: The Foreign Policy Centre in association with Clifford Chance).

Levin, L.S., McMahon, L. and Ziglio, E. (eds) (1994) *Economic Change, Social Welfare and Health in Europe* (Copenhagen: World Health Organisation Regional Office for Europe).

Lessof, R. and Figueras, J. (1998) 'Evidence for action: the European observatory on health care systems', *Eurohealth*, 4 (5), Winter: 33–5.

Lincoln, P., Doyle, N. and Pettersen, B. (1998) 'The new European public health framework (2000–2005): Implications for health promotion – an initial response', *Eurohealth*, 4 (5), Winter: 17–19.

Ludvigsen, C. and Roberts, K. (1996) *Health Care Policies and Europe: the Implications for Practice* (Oxford: Butterworth–Heinemann).

Lund, M. (1998) 'European health information today'. *Eurohealth*, 4 (1), Winter: 14–16.

Maarse, H. and van der Made, J. (1998) 'Cost containment and the right to health care', *European Journal of Public Health*, 8 (2): 119–26.

McCarthy, F.T. (1998) 'Shunned Nobel Prize Winner will Head new Research into BSE', *Daily Telegraph*, 8 June (London).

MacDonald, T.H. (1998) *Rethinking Health Promotion: A Global Approach* (London: Routledge).

Mackenbach, J.P. (1996) 'The history of public health in Europe', *European Journal of Public Health*, 6 (2): 79–80.

Mackenbach, J.P. and Kunst, A.E. (1999) 'Socioeconomic inequalities in health in Europe', *Eurohealth*, 5 (1), Spring: 31–4.

McKee, M. (1998a) 'Editorial: an agenda for public health research in Europe', *European Journal of Public Health*, 8 (1): 3–7.

McKee, M. (1998b) 'Does the WHO have a role in Europe?', *British Medical Journal*, 316, 9 May: 1402–3.

McKee, M. and Mossialos, E. (1997) 'Public health and European integration', in G. Scally (pp. 31–56.)

McKee, M., Mossialos, E. and Belcher, P. (1996) 'The Influence of European law on national health policy', *Journal of European Social Policy*, 6 (4): 263–86.

Mc Keown, T. (1979) *The Role of Medicine: Dream, Mirage or Nemesis?* (Oxford: Blackwell).

Maclay, M. (1998) *The European Union* (Stroud: Sutton Publishing).

Majone, G. (1996) 'A European regulatory state?' in J. Richardson pp. 263–77.

Majone, G. (1998) 'Understanding regulatory growth in the European Community' in D. Hine and K. Hussein (14–35.)

Malone, G. (1996) 'Minister of State – Department of Health UK – Summary of Presentation' in IMS International, *Round Table [One] 'Completing the Single Pharmaceutical Market' Proceedings* (Frankfurt am Main: IMS International in association with EFPIA and Pharmaceutical Partners for Better Health Care).

Markowe, H. (1999) 'Improving information for the development of public health', *Eurohealth*, 5 (1), Spring: 5–6.

Marris, P. (1996) *The Politics of Uncertainty: Attachment in Private and Public Life* (London: Routledge).

Maynard, A. (1999) 'Towards an integrated health care policy in the European Union?', *Eurohealth*, 5 (2), Summer: 5–6.

Maynard, A. and Bloor, K. (1995) 'Health care reform: informing difficult choices', *International Journal of Health Planning and Management*, 1 (4): 247–64.

Maynard, A. and Bloor, K. (1997) 'Regulating the pharmaceutical industry', *British Medical Journal*, 315, 26 July: 200–1.

Maynard, A. and Walker, A. (1997) *The Physician Workforce in the United Kingdom: Issues, Prospects and Policies* (London: Nuffield Trust).

Mazey, S. and Richardson, J. (1996) 'The logic of organisation: interest groups' in Richardson (1996), pp. 203–9.

Merkel, B. (1995) 'The public health competence of the European Community', *Eurohealth*, 1 (1), June: 21–2.

Meulders, D. and Plasman, R. (1997) 'European economic policies and social quality' in Beck *et al.*, pp. 19–39.

Michie, S. and Cockcroft, A. (1996) 'Overwork can kill', *British Medical Journal*, 312, 13 April: 921–2.

Mihill, C. (1995) 'Euro cancer list shows failings', *Guardian*, 17 May.

Milton, C. (1995) 'Survival rate below norm in British cancer cases', *The Times*, 17 May.

Moe, T. (1990) 'The politics of structural choice: toward a theory of public bureaucracy' in O.E. Williamson (ed.), *Organization Theory from Chester Barnard to the Present* (Oxford: Oxford University Press).

Morris, J.N. (1975) *Uses of Epidemiology, (3rd edn)* (Edinburgh: Churchill Livingstone).

Mossialos, E. (1996) 'Whither European pharmaceutical policy', *Eurohealth*, 2 (2), June: 16–17.

Mossialos, E. (1997) 'Citizens' views on health care systems in the 15 member states of the European Union', *Health Economics*, 6 (2): 109–16.

Mossialos, E. and McKee, M. (1997) 'The European Union and health: past, present and future' in A. Harrison, pp. 224–38.

Mossialos, E. and Le Grand, J. (eds) (1999) *Health Care and Cost Containment in the European Union* (Aldershot: Ashgate).

Mossialos, E. and McKee, M. (1998) 'The Amsterdam Treaty and the future of European health services', *Journal of Health Services Research and Policy*, 3 (2): 65–7.

Mossialos, E., McKee, M. and Rathwell, T. (1997c) 'Health care and the single market', *European Journal of Public Health*, 7 (3): 235–7.

Mossialos, E. and Permanand, G. (1998) 'A New European Commission: Wendezeit or Déjà Vu for Public Health?', *Eurohealth*, 4 (5), Winter: 1.

Mossialos, E., McKee, M., Rafferty, A-M. and Olsen, N. (1998) 'Editorial – a new chapter in public health: Britain's changing relationship with the European Union', *Journal of Epidemiology and Community Health*, 52 (10): 606–7.

Mountford, L. (1998a) 'European Union health policy on the eve of the millennium, – a working document produced by the Directorate General for Research for the European Parliament [Public Health and Consumer Protection Series – SACO 102 EN] (Luxembourg: European Parliament).

Mountford, L. (1998b) 'European Union health policy on the eve of the millennium', *Eurohealth*, 4 (5), Winter: 12–13.

Muntaner, C. and Lynch, J. (1999) 'Income inequality, social cohesion and class relations: a critique of Wilkinson's neo-Durkheimian research program', *International Journal of Health Services*, 29 (1): 59–81.

NAO (National Audit Office) (1998) *BSE: The Cost of a Crisis – Report by the Comptroller and Auditor General to the House of Commons (HC 853 Session 1997–98)* (London: The Stationery Office).

Neal, A.C. and Wright, F.B. (eds) (1992) *The European Communities' Health and Safety Legislation – Volume 1: The Social Dimension 1957–1991* (London: Chapman & Hall).

Needle, C. (1998) 'Developing public health in the EU', *Eurohealth*, 4 (3), Summer: 1998.

Newman, M. (1993) *The European Community – Where Does the Power Lie?* (European Dossier Series) (London: University of North London Press).

News EU (News from the European Union) (1995a) 'Notes', *Eurohealth*, 1 (2), October: 35.

News EU (News from the European Union) (1995b) 'Parliament strengthens health programmes – health promotion' and 'Health programmes go to conciliation', *Eurohealth*, 1 (3), December: 39, 41.

News EU (News from the European Union) (1996a) 'Meeting of EU health ministers', 'European health card' and 'Parliament strengthens health monitoring proposal', *Eurohealth*, 2 (2), June: 34, 35.

News EU (News from the European Union) (1996b) 'Parliament hearing on BSE/CJD', *Eurohealth*, 2 (3), September: 39.

News EU (News from the European Union) (1996c) 'Commission divided over contradictory tobacco policies' and 'Health funding attacked', *Eurohealth*, 2 (4), December: 39, 40.

News EU (News from the European Union) (1997a) 'Tobacco: health versus agriculture' and 'Health, poverty and exclusion: European conference to encourage international cooperation', *Eurohealth*, 3 (1), Spring: 43, 45.

News EU (News from the European Union) (1997b) 'Action programme against pollution-related illness', 'Reducing accidents and injuries' and 'A community action programme for rare diseases', *Eurohealth*, 3 (2), Summer: 47, 48.

News EU (News from the European Union (1997c) 'Free movement and pharmaceutical patents', 'Free movement of patients' and 'Accidents in the workplace', *Eurohealth*, 3 (3), Autumn: 39, 40.

News EU (News from the European Union (1998a) 'Health council', 'Frankfurt Round Table on pharmaceuticals' and 'European health and safety at work report', *Eurohealth*, 4 (1), Winter: 38.

News EU (News from the European Union) (1998b) 'Commissioner Flynn addresses meeting of the Health Intergroup', 'Tobacco remains a burning issue' and 'European Parliament Plenary Session – Strasbourg, March 9–13', *Eurohealth*, 4 (2), Spring: 39, 40, 41.

News EU (News from the European Union) (1998c) 'Free movement of medical practitioners', 'Health Council meeting', 'Boosting competitiveness for the pharmaceutical sector', 'Commission website on pharmaceuticals' and 'Agreement on disease surveillance network', *Eurohealth*, 4 (3), Summer: 45, 47, 48, 49.

News EU (News from the European Union) (1998d) 'Eurostat publishes findings on accidents in the workplace' and 'Towards increased harmonisation of Member State health systems?', *Eurohealth*, 4 (4), Autumn: 44, 45.

News EU (News from the European Union) (1999a) 'Flynn specifies Commission competencies in health', 'Commission agrees 1999 programme against drug abuse', 'Parliament reiterates its positions on rare and pollution-linked diseases', 'BSE – Mixed Results', 'UK ban lifted' and 'Health Council Meeting, Brussels', *Eurohealth*, 4 (5), Winter: 37, 38, 39, 40, 41.

News EU (News from the European Union) (1999b) 'Further agreement on injury prevention', 'Agreement on rare diseases and pollution-related diseases', 'Brutland calls for increased WHO–EU co-operation' and 'News in Brief', *Eurohealth*, 5 (1), Spring: 50, 51, 52.

News EU (News from the European Union) (1999c) 'Stop Press – 3 June – Prodi Announces New Commission DG for Health', 'Meeting of the High Level Committee on Health' and 'News in brief', *Eurohealth*, 5 (2), Summer: 42, 43, 44.

Nielsen, R. and Szyszczak, E. (1997) *The Social Dimension of the European Union 3rd edn* (Copenhagen: Handelshøjskolens Forlag).

Nickless, A.J. (1999) 'Kohll and Decker: a new hope for third-country nationals', *Eurohealth*, 5 (1), Spring: 20–2.

Norris, P. (1998) 'The impact of European harmonisation on Norwegian drug policy', *Health Policy*, 43: 65–81.

Nugent, N. (1994) *The Government and Politics of the European Union (3rd edn)* (London: Macmillan).

Nugent, N. (ed.) (1997) *At the Heart of the Union: Studies of the European Commission* (London: Macmillan).

OECD (1994) *The Reform of Health Care Systems: a Review of Seventeen OECD Countries* (Health Policy Studies No. 5) (Paris: OECD).

OECD (1996) (Organisation for Economic Co-operation and Development) *Health Data 95* (Paris: OECD).

OECD (1998) *Labour Market and Social Policy – Occasional Papers No. 33 – Social and Health Policies in OECD countries: A Survey of Current Programmes and Recent*

Developments – DEELSA/ELSA/WD(98)4 (written for the OECD by David W. Kalisch, Tetsuya Aman and Libbie A. Buchele) (Paris: OECD).

OECD (1999) *Labour Market and Social Policy – Occasional Papers No. 36 – Health Outcomes in OECD Countries: a Framework of Health Indicators for Outcome-Oriented Policymaking – DEELSA/ELSA/WD(98)7* (written by Melissa Jee and Zeynep Or) (Paris: OECD).

OHE (Office of Health Economics) (1982) *Ill in Europe (OHE Briefing No. 20, October)* (London: Office of Health Economics).

OJ (*Official Journal of the European Communities*) (1965) 'Council Directive 65/65/ EEC of 26 January 1965 on the approximation of provisions laid down by law, regulation or administrative action relating to medicinal products', OJL No. 22 of 9-2-65, p. 369 (Luxembourg: Office for Official Publications of the European Communities) [Subsequently amended by Directives 66/454/EEC, 75/319/EEC, 83/570/EEC, 87/21/EEC, 87/21/EEC, 89/341/EEC, 89/342/EEC, 89/343/EEC, 92/ 27/EEC, 92/73/EEC and 93/39/EEC].

OJ (*Official Journal of the European Communities*) (1979) 'Council Directive 79/112/ EEC on the approximation of the laws of Member States relating to the labelling, presentation and advertising of foodstuffs for sale to the ultimate consumer', *OJ*, L033 08/02/79.

OJ (*Official Journal of the European Communities*) (1987) 'The Europe against cancer programme, proposals by the European Commission', *OJ*, No. C 50 of 26/2/87.

OJ (*Official Journal of the European Communities*) (1990) 'Decision of the Council and representatives of the government of Member States meeting in the Council, adopting an action plan 1990–1994 in the framework of the Europe against cancer programme', *OJ*, L 137 of 30/5/90.

OJ (*Official Journal of the European Communities*) (1992) 'Council Directive 92/59/ EEC on general product safety', *OJ*, L228 of 11/08/92.

OJ (*Official Journal of the European Communities*) (1993) 'Council Regulation (EEC) No. 2309/93 of 22 July establishing EMEA', *OJ*, EC L 214 of 24/8/1993 (Luxembourg: Office for Official Publications of the European Communities).

OJ (*Official Journal of the European Communities*) (1994) 'Proposal for a European Parliament and Council Decision adopting a programme of Community action on the prevention of drug dependence within the framework for action in the field of public health (1995–2000)', *OJ*, 94/C 257/04. (Luxembourg: Office for Official Publications of the European Communities).

OJ (*Official Journal of the European Communities*) (1995) 'European Parliament and Council Decision No. 1729/95/EC of 19 June 1995 on the extension of the "Europe against AIDS" programme', *OJ*, L 1995/168-2EN.

OJ (*Official Journal of the European Communities* (1996) 'Decision No. 646/96/EC of the European Parliament and the Council of 29 March 1996 adopting an action plan to combat cancer within the framework for action in the field of public health (1996 to 2000)', *OJ*, L 1996/95-3EN.

OJ (*Official Journal of the European Communities*) (1999) 'Decision No. 283/1999/EC of the European Parliament and the Council of 25 January establishing a general framework for Community activities in favour of consumers', *OJ*, L 1999/34-7EN.

Osborne, D. and Gaebler, T. (1993) *Reinventing Government* (London: Plume-Penguin Books).

Parker, G., Maitland, A., Southey, C. and Kampfner J. (1996) 'Older dairy cows face slaughter' and 'Food crisis may blight European summit', *The Financial Times*, 27 March: 1.

Partridge, Sir M., Moodie, M. and the ACE Working Group (1998) *The Partridge Enquiry: Report by the Ace Working Group on Social Europe: Risk or Opportunity?* (London: Action Centre for Europe Ltd).

Pedersen, S. (1999) 'Telemedicine in the Future' in. Wootton and Craig, pp. 191–5.

Peters, B.G. (1994) 'Agenda-setting in the European Community', *Journal of European Public Policy*, 1 (1): 9–26.

Petersen, A. and Lupton, D. (1996) *The New Public Health: Health and Self in the Age of Risk* (London: Sage).

Peterson, J. and Bomberg, E. (1999) *Decision-Making in the European Union* (London: Macmillan).

Phillips Inquiry (Inquiry into BSE – Chairman Sir Nicholas Phillips) (1998-) – see Inquiry web site http://www.bse.org.uk/ which contains numerous working documents and transcripts of evidence given and a fact file containing key dates and information.

Pidgeon, N., Henwood, K. and Horlick-Jones, T. (1999) 'Risk communication: new challenges for European health policy', *Eurohealth*, 5 (2), Summer: 12–14.

Pierson, P. (1996) 'The path for European intergration: a historical institutionalist analysis; *Comparative Political Studies*, 2a (2), April: 123–63.

Piha, T. (1999) 'Tackling health determinants through health promotion and disease prevention', *Eurohealth*, 5 (1), Spring: 7–8.

Pinder, J. (1998) *The Building of the European Union, (3rd edn)* (Oxford: Oxford University Press).

Putnam, R.D. (1993) *Making Democracy Work: Civic Traditions in Modern Italy* (Princeton: Princeton University Press).

Putnam, R.D. (1995) 'Tuning in, tuning out: the strange disappearance of social capital in America', *Political Science and Politics*, December: 664–83.

Putters, K. and van der Grinten, T. (1998) 'Health impact screening: the administrative function of a health policy instrument', *Eurohealth*, 4 (3), Summer: 29–31.

Rajala, M. (1998) 'The European Commission's activities in the field of health promotion', *Eurohealth*, 4 (5): 14–16.

Ranade, W. (1997) *A Future for the NHS? Health Care for the Millennium, 2nd edn* (Harlow: Longman).

Randall, E. (1997) 'Health policy and the European Union', in Symes *et al.* pp. 272–98.

Ratzan, S.C. (ed.) (1998) *The Mad Cow Crisis: Health and the Public Good* (London: UCL Press).

Reiner, Z. (1998) 'WHO and the EU: united will they stand?', *Eurohealth*, 4 (6), Special Issue – Winter: 2–4.

REITOX (The European Information Network on Drugs and Drug Addiction) [a network of National Focal Points (NFPs) set up in the 15 EU Member States and the European Commission, and an observer Focal Point in Norway, along with EMCDDA it acts as a practical instrument for the exchange of data and information] web address http://www.emcdda.org/html/reitox.html (Lisbon).

Rhodes, M. (1995) 'A regulatory conundrum: industrial relations and the social dimension' in Leibfried and Pierson, pp. 78–122.

Richards, T. (ed.) (1992) *Medicine in Europe* (London: *British Medical Journal*).

Richards, T. (1997) Editorial 'Europe Matters – and doctors should get involved', *British Medical Journal*, 314, 15 February: 460.

Richards, T. (1999) 'European observatory will promote better health policy – Tessa Richards speaks to Josep Figueras, co-ordinator of the Observatory's activities', *British Medical Journal*, 318, 6 February: 352.

Richardson, J. (ed.) (1996) *European Union: Power and Policy-Making* (London: Routledge).

RIIA (Royal Institute of International Affairs, The) (1997) *An Equal Partner: Britain's Role in a Changing Europe – Final Report on Britain and Europe* (London: The Royal Institute of International Affairs).

Rodgers, A. (1999) 'The European Commission, risk management and the precautionary principle', *Eurohealth*, 5 (2), Summer: 15–18.

Rogers, A. (1996) 'European Union's role in public health unsettled', *Lancet*, 347, 20 April: 1107.

Room, G. (ed.) (1991) *Towards a European Welfare State?* (Bristol: SAUS Publications).

Rosenmöller, M. (1998) 'Enlargement of the European Union: challenges for health and health care', *Eurohealth*, 4 (4), Autumn: 18–21.

Rosenmöller, M (1999) 'EU enlargement – the influence on the EU health agenda', *Eurohealth*, 5 (1), Spring: 11.

Ross, G. (1995) *Jacques Delors and European Integration* (Cambridge: Policy Press in association with Blackwell Publishers).

Roth-Behrendt, D. (1998) 'From BSE to a new EU food and consumer health policy: European Parliament's role as a catalyst for change', *Eurohealth*, 4 (2), Spring: 2–3.

Saltman, R.B. (1997) 'Equity and distributive justice in European health care reform', *International Journal of Health Services*, 27 (3): 443–53.

Saltman, R.B. and Figueras, J. (1997) *European Health Care Reform: Analysis of Current Strategies* (Copenhagen: World Health Organisation).

Saltman, R.B., Figueras, J. and Sakellarides, C (eds) (1998) *Critical Challenges for Health Care Reform in Europe* (Buckingham: Open University Press).

Sandholtz, W. and Stone Sweet A. (eds) (1998) *European Integration and Supranational Governance* (Oxford: Oxford University Press).

Sandman, P.M. (1999) 'Mass media and environmental risk: seven principles' in R. Bate (1999) *What Risk? Science, Politics & Public Health* (revised paperback edition) (Oxford: Butterworth–Heinemann).

Santer, J. (1997) 'Speech by Jacques Santer – President of the European Commission in response to the Debate in the European Parliament on the report by the Committee of Inquiry into BSE', Commission Press Release, SPEECH/97/39 (Brussels).

Sassi, F. (1996) 'Health technology assessment – an introduction', *Eurohealth*, 2 (4): 9–10.

Sauer, F. (1992) 'The European Community's pharmaceutical policy', in Hermans *et al.* (1992)

Sauer, F. (1998) 'European Medicines Evaluation Agency is ahead of national licensing authorities – Letters', *British Medical Journal*, 317, 17 October: 1078.

SCADPlus European Union web-based guide to Union Policies with a comprehensive policy index at http://europa.eu.int/scadplus/leg/en/l00000.htm (provides information on almost all the policy areas with which the Commission is concerned and includes brief presentations of Commission proposals together with details of their progress up to their final adoption. Further information is provided in background notes, which help to explain the development and future prospects of legislative work relating to Community policies).

Scally, G. (ed.) (1997) *Progress in Public Health* (London: The Royal Society of Medicine Press).

Schofield, R. and Shaoul, J. 'E.coli 0157: public health vs private wealth', *Eurohealth*, 4 (4), Autumn: 34–7.

SEAC (Spongiform Encephalopathy Advisory Committee) (1998) *SEAC Annual Report 1997–1998* (http://www.maff.gov.uk/maffhome.htm).

SEAC (Spongiform Encephalopathy Advisory Committee) (1999) *SEAC Annual Report for 1998–1999* (http://www.maff.gov.uk/maffhome.htm).

Sheldon, T. (1993) 'Vive la difference?', *Health Services Journal*, 15 July.

Simpson, R. and Walker R. (eds) (1993) *Europe: For Richer or Poorer?* (London: Child Poverty Action Group).

Sissouras, A. (1998) 'Establishing health monitoring systems in Europe', *Eurohealth*, 4 (5), Winter: 9–11.

Smith, D.J. (1980) *Overseas Doctors in the National Health Service* (London: Policy Studies Institute).

Smith, R. (1987) *Unemployment and Health: a Disaster and a Challenge* (Oxford: Oxford University Press).

Smith, R. (1997) 'The future of healthcare systems: information technology and consumerism will transform health care worldwide', *British Medical Journal*, 314, 24 May: 1495.

Smith, T. (1991) 'Joining Europe: closer links with Europe may improve standards of health care in Britain', *British Medical Journal*, 303, 23 November: 1284.

Smith, T. (1992) 'European health challenges', in T. Richards (pp. 13–22.)

Southey, C. (1996) 'BSE scare prompts ill feeling in Brussels', *The Financial Times*, 27 March: 9.

Sosa-Iudicissa, M. (ed.) (1996) *Final Report 3rd Framework Programme Telematics Systems for Health Care (AIM) 1991–1994 Volumes 1 & 2* (Brussels – European Commission – DGXIII).

Stacey, M. (1995) 'The British General Medical Council: from Empire to Europe' in Johnson *et al.*, pp. 116–38.

Stallknect, K. (1992) 'Nursing in Europe', in T. Richards, (59–64.)

Stein, H. (1995) 'Experiences of the German Presidency: small steps towards integrating public health', *Eurohealth*, 1 (1), June: 19–20.

Stein, H. (1996) 'Public health and public health research – the need for concerted action at European Union level', *Eurohealth*, 2 (2), June: 23–4.

Stein, H. (1997) 'The Treaty of Amsterdam & Article 129: a second chance for public health in Europe' and 'Future framework for public health', *Eurohealth*, 3 (2), Summer: 4–8.

Stein, H. (1998) 'Euro health 2000: a missed opportunity. comments on the Commission Communication on the development of public health policy in the European Community', *Eurohealth*, 4 (5), Winter: 5–8.

Stewart, A. (1999) 'Cost-containment and privatization: an international analysis' in Drache and Sullivan, 65–84.

Stirk, P.M.R. and Weigall, D. (eds) (1999) *The Origins and Development of European Integration: a reader and Commentary* (London: Pinter).

Stöhr, K. with Crom, R.L., Meslin, F-X. and Heymann, D.L. (1998) 'The public health impact of the Use of antimicrobials in food animals', *Eurohealth*, 4 (2), Spring: 7–9.

Stone Sweet, A. and Caporaso, J.A. (1998) 'From free trade to supranational policy: the European court and integration' in Sandholtz and Stone Sweet, pp. 92–133.

Symes, V., Levy, C. and Littlewood, J. (eds) (1997) *The Future of Europe: Problems and Issues for the Twenty-First Century* (London: Macmillan).

Taylor, D. (1992) 'Prescribing in Europe – Forces for Change', in Richards, pp. 91–100.

Taylor, D. (1997) 'Patently confused', *British Medical Journal*, 314, 3 May: 1296.

Taylor, D. and Maynard, A. (1990) *Medicines, the NHS and Europe: Balancing the Public's Interests*, briefing paper II (London: King's Fund Institute in association with The Centre for Health Economics University of York).

Teeling-Smith, G. (ed.) (1989) *Measuring the Benefits of Medicines: the Future Agenda* (London: Office of Health Economics).

Ter Kuile, B.H. (1992) 'Introduction', in Hermans *et al.*, pp. 1–2.

Tiemann, F. (1999) 'Reacting rapidly to threats to health', *Eurohealth*, 5 (1), Spring: 6–7.

Townsend, J. (1991) 'Tobacco and the European common agricultural policy: European gold kills', *British Medical Journal*, 303, 26 October: 1008–9.

Townsend, P. (1992) *Hard Times: the Prospects for European Social Policy* (Eleanor Rathbone Memorial Lecture given on 4 March 1991) (Liverpool: Liverpool University Press).

Townsend, P. and Davidson, N. and Whitehead, M. (1992) *Inequalities in Health: The Black Report* and the *Health Divide* – new edition updated and revised (London: Penguin Books).

Tremblay, M. (1993) *Health Policy and Europe: an Introduction to Some of the Issues (Discussion Paper 31)* (Birmingham: Health Services Management Centre – The University of Birmingham).

Turner, J. (1995) 'What Ken Collins has to say', *Eurohealth*, 1 (1), June: 10–11.

UN (United Nations) (1995) *Copenhagen Declaration* (World Summit for Social Development) (available on world wide web http://www.webonly.com/socdev/wssd.htm) (UN/Division for Social Policy and Development).

Unwin, Sir B., (1999) 'Financing healthcare capital investment: the role of the European Investment Bank', *Eurohealth*, 5 (2), Summer: 7–8.

Usher, J.A. (1998) *EC Institutions and Legislation* (Harlow: Longman).

van der Mei, A.P. (1999) 'The Kohll and Decker rulings: revolution of evolution?', *Eurohealth*, 5 (1), Spring: 14–16.

van de Water, H.P.A., Perenboom, R.J.M. and Boshuizen, H.C. (1996) 'Policy relevance of the health expectancy indicator: an inventory in European countries', *Health Policy*, 36: 117–29.

Veil, S. (1997) *Report of the High Level Panel on the Free Movement of Persons – (Presented to the Commission on 18 March)* (Luxembourg: Office for Official Publications of the European Communities).

Viegas, S.F. and Dunn, K. (eds) (1998) *Telemedicine: Practicing in the Information Age* (Philadelphia: Lippincott-Raven).

Vos, E. (1999) *Institutional Frameworks of Community Health & Safety Regulation: Committees, Agencies and Private Bodies* (Oxford: Hart Publishing).

Wallace, H. and Wallace, W. (eds) (1996) *Policy-Making in the European Union* (Oxford: Oxford University Press).

Watson, Rodger (1999) 'A blueprint for Europe', *Nursing Standard*, 13 (18), 20–6 January: 25–6.

Watson, Rory (1994a) 'Meddling or benefiting: health in Europe?', *British Medical Journal*, 308, 1 January: 12.

Watson, Rory (1994b) 'Blood is a European issue', *British Medical Journal*, 309, 29 October: 1110.

Watson, Rory (1995) 'How Eurocrats affect our health', *British Medical Journal*, 311, 29 July: 282.

Watson, Rory (1998) 'EU attempts to tackle parallel pricing of drugs', *British Medical Journal*, 316, 13 June: 1769.

Watson, Rory (1999a) 'News – European Commission proposes public health department', *British Medical Journal*, 318, 3 April: 893.

Watson, Rory (1999b) 'News – EU tackles pollution related illness', *British Medical Journal*, 318, 8 May: 1234.

Watson, Rory (1999c) 'EU says growth hormones pose health risk', *British Medical Journal*, 318, 29 May: 1442.

Watson, Rory (1999d) 'European Union considers new plan to help refugees', *British Medical Journal*, 318, 29 May: 1439.

Weale, A. (1994) 'Social policy and the European Union', *Social Policy and Administration*, 28 (1), March: 5–19.

Weil, O. and McKee, M. (1998) 'Setting priorities for health in Europe: are we speaking the same language?', *European Journal of Public Health*, 8 (3): 256–8.

Wells, N. (1980) *Medicines: 50 Years of Progress 1930–1980* (London: Office of Health Economics).

Wendon, B. (1998) 'The Commission as image-venue entrepreneur in EU social policy', *Journal of European Public Policy*, 5 (2): 339–53.

Whitehead, M. and Dahlgren, G. (1994) 'Editorial – why not now?: Action on inequalities in health', *European Journal of Public Health*, 4 (1): 1–2.

Whitehead, M. (1998) 'Diffusion of ideas on social inequalities in health: a European perspective', *Milbank Quarterly*, 76 (3): 469–92.

WHO (World Health Organization) (1978) *Declaration of Alma-Ata* (Copenhagen: Regional Office for Europe).

WHO (World Health Organization) (1981) *Global Strategy for Health for All by the Year 2000* (Copenhagen: WHO Regional Office for Europe).

WHO (World Health Organization) (1986) *Ottawa Charter for Health Promotion* (Copenhagen: WHO Regional Office for Europe).

WHO (World Health Organization) (1990) *The Milan Declaration on Healthy Cities* (Copenhagen: WHO Regional Office for Europe).

WHO (World Health Organization) (1994a) *Helsinki Declaration for Action of Environment and Health in Europe* (Copenhagen: WHO Regional Office for Europe).

WHO (World Health Organization) (1994b) *The Copenhagen Declaration* (Copenhagen: WHO Regional Office for Europe).

WHO (World Health Organization) (1996) *The Ljubljana Charter on Reforming Health Care* (Copenhagen: WHO Regional Office for Europe).

WHO (World Health Organization) (1998a) *Athens Declaration for Healthy Cities* (Copenhagen: WHO Regional Office for Europe).

WHO (World Health Organization) Regional Office for Europe (1998b) *Health in Europe 1997* (Copenhagen: WHO Regional Office for Europe).

WHO (World Health Organisation) (1998c) *A Heath Telematics Policy* (document DGO/98.1) (Geneva: WHO).

Wilkinson, R.G. (1996) *Unhealthy Societies: the Afflictions of Inequality* (London: Routledge).

Wiley, M.W. (1995) 'Hospital financing in Europe', *Eurohealth*, 1 (1), June: 23–4.

Wise, M. and Gibb, R. (1993) *Single Market to Social Europe: The European Community in the 1990s* (Harlow: Longman Scientific & Technical with John Wiley).

Wold-Olsen, P. (1998) 'A single market for pharmaceuticals: from contradiction to reality', *Eurohealth*, 4 (2), Spring: 22–4.

Wootton, R. and Craig, J. (eds) (1999) *Introduction to Telemedicine* (London: The Royal Society of Medicine Press).

Index

Abbasi, Kamran, 87
Abel-Smith, Brian, 26, 28, 159, 173, 174
Abrahamson, Peter, 192
accidents and injuries, 24, 33, 121, 123–5
Acheson, Sir Donald, 141, 192, 193, 207, 235
Acquired Immunodeficiency Syndrome (AIDS), 20, 24, 102–5
adaptability and EU policy, 211
Adenaur, Konrad, 5
Advanced Informatics in Medicine (AIM), 163–4, 177
Advisory Committee for Safety, Hygiene and Health Protection at Work (ACSHH), 35, 37–8, 40, 41–2
Advisory Committee on Medical Training, 62
Advisory Committee on Training in Nursing, 62
ageing population, 18
Agenda 2000, 28–9
AIDS, *see* Acquired Immunodeficiency Syndrome
Alma Ata Declaration, 8
Amsterdam, Treaty of, *see* Treaty of Amsterdam
Andersen Consulting, 188
animal feed, 140–1, 144, 145, 146
antibiotic resistance, 126
anti-poverty policy, an EU, 217
Arrow, Kenneth, 77
Ashton, John, 10
Association of Schools of Public Health in the European Region (ASPHER), 14, 118, 119
Athens Declaration on Healthy Cities, 8
Atkinson, Tony, 215, 216–18

Baggott, Rob, 17–18
Bainbridge, Timothy add in
Bangemann, Martin, 75, 77
Barber, Lionel, 64

basic income schemes, 218
BBC (British Broadcasting Corporation), 156
Bean, Charles, 193, 214, 219
beef ban, EU Commission, 144, 148, 152, 153
beggar-my-neighbour policies, 219
Belcher, Paul, 6, 14, 95, 159
Belgium, 82, 224
Ben-Shlomo, Yoav, 191
Bentolila, Samuel, 193
Benzeval, Michaela, 193
Berlin, A., 52
Bertola, Guiseppe, 193
Beveridge, William, 4, 5
Bilbao, 43, 45, 226
BIOMED (Biomedical and Health Research Programme of the EU), 104
biomolecular revolution, 138
Blair, Tony, 101, 178
Blane, David, 191
blood safety, 125
Bloor, Karen, 175
Bomberg, Elizabeth, 132
Bolivia, 108
Bovine Spongiform Encephalopathy, *see* BSE
breast cancer, 98, 99
Britain, *see* United Kingdom
British Medical Association (BMA), 113, 138
British Medical Journal (BMJ), 40, 50, 65, 87–8
British Pharmaceutical Price Regulation Scheme (PPRS), *see* pharmaceutical industry
Brussels, 49, 72, 113, 122, 128, 131, 132, 209
BSE, xi, 14, 20, 24–5, 137–58, 224
    impact on EU politics, 139–40
    origins of, 140–1
    puzzling disease, a, 141–2

278   *Index*